A CULTURAL HISTORY
OF MEDICINE

VOLUME 6

A Cultural History of Medicine
General Editor: Roger Cooter

Volume 1
A Cultural History of Medicine in Antiquity
Edited by Laurence Totelin

Volume 2
A Cultural History of Medicine in the Middle Ages
Edited by Iona McCleery

Volume 3
A Cultural History of Medicine in the Renaissance
Edited by Elaine Leong and Claudia Stein

Volume 4
A Cultural History of Medicine in the Enlightenment
Edited by Lisa Wynne Smith

Volume 5
A Cultural History of Medicine in the Age of Empire
Edited by Jonathan Reinarz

Volume 6
A Cultural History of Medicine in the Modern Age
Edited by Todd Meyers

A CULTURAL HISTORY OF MEDICINE

IN THE MODERN AGE

Edited by Todd Meyers

BLOOMSBURY ACADEMIC
LONDON • NEW YORK • OXFORD • NEW DELHI • SYDNEY

BLOOMSBURY ACADEMIC
Bloomsbury Publishing Plc
50 Bedford Square, London, WC1B 3DP, UK
1385 Broadway, New York, NY 10018, USA
29 Earlsfort Terrace, Dublin 2, Ireland

BLOOMSBURY, BLOOMSBURY ACADEMIC and the Diana logo are trademarks
of Bloomsbury Publishing Plc

First published in Great Britain 2021
This paperback edition first published 2024

Copyright © Bloomsbury Publishing, 2021

Todd Meyers has asserted his right under the Copyright, Designs and Patents Act, 1988,
to be identified as Editor of this work.

Cover image © Wellcome Library, London

A catalogue record for this book is available from the British Library.

Library of Congress Cataloging-in-Publication Data
Names: Cooter, Roger, editor.
Title: A cultural history of medicine / general editor, Roger Cooter.
Description: London ; New York : Bloomsbury Academic, 2021. |
Series: The cultural histories series | Includes bibliographical references and index. |
Identifiers: LCCN 2020051490 | ISBN 9781472569936 (hardback)
Subjects: LCSH: Medicine–History.
Classification: LCC R131 .C78 2021 | DDC 610.9—dc23
LC record available at https://lccn.loc.gov/2020051490

ISBN: HB: 978-1-4725-6988-2
       Set: 978-1-4725-6987-5
       PB: 978-1-3504-5162-9
       Set: 978-1-3504-5164-3

Series: The Cultural Histories Series

Typeset by RefineCatch Limited, Bungay, Suffolk
Printed and bound in Great Britain

To find out more about our authors and books visit www.bloomsbury.com
and sign up for our newsletters.

CONTENTS

ILLUSTRATIONS

INTRODUCTION

CHAPTER 1

CHAPTER 2

CHAPTER 7

CHAPTER 8

GENERAL EDITOR'S PREFACE

ROGER COOTER

The cultural history of medicine is all embracing. Virtually nothing can be excluded from it – the body in all its literary and other representations over time, ideas of civilization and humankind, and the sociology, anthropology and epistemology of health and welfare, not to mention the existential experiences of pain, disease, suffering and death, and the way professionals have endeavoured to deal with them. To contain much of this vastness, the volumes in this series focus on eight categories, all of contemporary relevance: environment, food, disease, animals, objects, experience, mind/brain and authority. From the ancient through to the postmodern world, these themes are pursued with critical breadth, depth and novelty by dedicated experts. Transnational perspectives are widely entertained. Above all these volumes attend to and illuminate what exactly is a *cultural* history of medicine, a category of investigation and an epistemological concept that has its emergence in the 1980s.

Introduction

TODD MEYERS

There is an inclination on the part of editors to begin the introduction to a volume by explaining to readers what the collection of essays is not doing – to define what is present by what is omitted or wholly absent. I share this tendency, but in this case I do so for a specific reason. To appreciate the cultural history of medicine in the past century (and I will come back to the first word in this phrase, 'cultural', in a moment, though 'history' requires some qualification as well), from the moments immediately after the First World War and the Spanish Flu to the era of AIDS and Ebola, requires us to acknowledge the historiography of the history of medicine within this otherwise arbitrary chronological frame. The writing of the history of medicine in the twentieth century – the priorities, sensibilities and different foci of this effort – is itself one culture, and one that has been cultivated most visibly by Anglophone, Francophone and Germanophone scholars.

Second, to appreciate the cultural history of medicine in the past century would require us to consider some uncomfortable 'where' questions – not only how broad or narrow the geographic horizon of this frame hopes or needs to be, but to consider what kinds of political and social unevenness is found there (Hunt, 1999; Fanon, 1994 [1965]; Farmer, 1992). That said, the effort of this volume is not without precedent. At different points over the past century, scholars have written and collated the history of medicine's history by accounting for transformations and innovations (both in medical science and the writing about it) across a jagged landscape (Braunstein, 2010; King, 1991; Iggers, 1997). And, unsurprisingly, there is an overwhelming body of scholarship that would otherwise put sweeping claims of steady progress on strident epistemological notice. Here I am thinking of work by Henry E. Sigerist (2018; 1994; 1960), Erwin Ackerknecht (1955), George Rosen (2015; 1949) and

Georges Canguilhem (2012), and later Roy Porter (2006; 1997), Charles Rosenberg (2007; 1998), Nancy Tomes (1998), Rosemary Stevens (1998; 1989) and Paul Starr (1984), and more recently (and with considerable overlap with the previous set of names) George Weisz (2014; 2005), Susan E. Lederer (1997), Andrea Tone (2001), Ilana Löwy (2011) and the general editor of this series, Roger Cooter (2013; 2007), to name but a few. Returning to my first point, this volume does not seek to reproduce or even mirror the incredible work of historians of medicine *in* the past century *of* the past century. Rather, the aim and approach here are quite different. The authors in the volume instead have chosen distinctive vantage points within this period, through the set of themes engaged in all six volumes of this series – different hilltops whereby to gain perspectives that allow them to comment in specific ways on cases not meant to be so much illustrative as they are evocative, still keeping each other in view, to conjure concepts and ideas that expose the culture of medicine in the twentieth century in unique though (as will become clear) complementary ways.

The culture of medicine in the twentieth century runs parallel to the history of public health and its cultural (indeed, global) reach (Packard, 2016). It is easy for one to cross into this other land without ever realizing it, and for good reason. It does not require careful scholarship or even that much cultural awareness to see how medicine and public health science move in tandem from a picture of disease as a wholly external threat to a history of disease and disorder bound up with human activity and human lack, forever compelled by social-political circumstances and real-felt connectedness. At the risk of generalization, medicine in all its valences has responded to the threat of disease and disorder through the promise to its own innovation, through its inexorable commitment to novel therapeutics (pharmacological, technical, behavioural), and by the dominance of its organizational and institutional capital (Porter, 1999). Medicine as an ideology finds its way into seemingly everything (Rose, 2007), with favourable (Porter, 1997) or corrosive (Illich, 1976) results. And at the risk of hyperbole, in the twentieth century, medicine finds the full expression of its self-awareness (as do its historians, particularly in relation to geopolitics, as the correspondence between Sigerist and such figures as Welch, Cushing, Garrison and Ackerknecht shows [2010]), something that happens at an early point in the century. A period of medical 'modernism' slipping into a 'post-modern' period is one in which medicine and its actors uncover and undertake an inventory of medicine's places and priorities, its imaginaries, its ambitions, its challenges and, unsurprisingly, its failures. The metaphor of man heroically pitted against disease fades, or at the very least begins to incorporate some awareness of shortcoming in that activity: the twentieth century finds medicine increasingly pitted against itself in its ideals (Tomes, 1998). AIDS, as one of many examples (though perhaps none so powerful), certainly invited new metaphors for the tripartite relationship of medicine, society and disease in the later part of the century (Fee and Fox, 1988; Treichler, 1999). AIDS created an opening, a dark lens for seeing problems and a blueprint for a question at the core of medical concern ever since: what is required of medicine when it encounters new domains of suffering, and how does medicine account for scale, population and power when these new areas of socio-medical concern emerge? It is much easier to predict the past than to be accountable to the present (though many have made careers doing just that). Still, what directions do we assume that medicine and cultural history of medicine have taken, seen from where we sit now, as they seek to establish new (and renewed) relationships between themselves and their objects (disease, patient, society), established seemingly anew again and again?

After assembling these chapters, I wonder if the so-called postmodern perspective within the cultural history of medicine of the twentieth century is how we are to understand ourselves or our particular point of view – if it is enough to simply strive for an accounting of where we are now, with a special emphasis on *where* (Golinski, 1998). Perhaps just as unsatisfying is a perspective that depends on some notion of pluralism (many cultures of this cultural history of medicine) (Burke, 2004). Is it a history that happens in other places, with other people (Biehl and Petryna, 2015; Livingston, 2012; Worsley, 1982), or one that is intimate, 'our' own history (Fee, 1983; Martin, 1987), however one defines these proximities or uses possessive pronouns? If a cultural history of medicine in the twentieth century offers anything, it is a picture of medicine that would only partially recognize itself in the image, not so much as a postmodern undertaking meant to undermine its value or power, but a psychodynamic exercise aimed at understanding itself in relation to the representation of itself – one that welcomes an image of medicine that is self-critical, technically-specific, contradictory, ethically tested, disarming, innovative, sometimes heroic, necessary and, most of all, experienced.

In this final volume of 'A Cultural History of Medicine', the chapters explore the ways in which biomedicine was organized through the regulation of the profession, how biomedicine responded unequally to challenges of new and re-emerging diseases, recognized disorder, ushered in new modes of therapy and classification, and reformed the cultures of medical practice and patienthood (Good, 1994; Porter, 1985). Each of the chapters places biomedicine in cultural perspective in terms of both geographic locale and a specific milieu of concepts and practices. In what follows, I offer a brief outline of each of the chapters and attempt to highlight the links between them. As I have already said, after placing these chapters side by side, it seems that their function as a cultural history of biomedicine between the modern and postmodern eras is, in part, an effort to consider the historiography of medical history itself, as a way of recognizing the interpretation of medical priorities and challenges across place and time, while attending to the particularities of specific cases (*case method* being something else decidedly twentieth century) (Forrester, 2017). It strikes me that what is so fundamental about the term 'medicine' or even 'biomedicine' in the twentieth

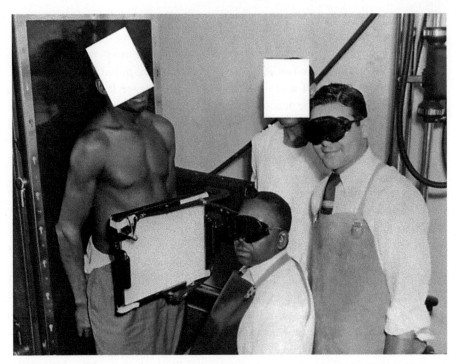

FIGURE 0.1: African-American man being x-rayed in the Tuskegee Study of Untreated Syphilis in the Negro Male, 1932. Credit: Gado Images / Alamy Stock Photo.

century is that it comes to stand for so many things at once: the practitioner, the clinic, the hospital (Adams, 2007), the profession of medicine as well as other allied professions, diagnostic practices (including the technologies to aid them), campaigns of disease control, an arbitrator of illness experience, a site of innovation and sometimes violence, a body of collective knowledge about healing, a point of contrast to an ethos of *vis medicatrix naturae* – and the list goes on. And just as there are seldom neat breaks in time within medical history, there are hazy borders between these versions of the 'medicine' as such. The following chapters move in and between these borders.

It needs to be said from the outset that this volume has not aimed to be exhaustive and the contributors have not attempted to produce an inventory of medicine and its instantiations (discoveries, controversies) of the last century. Again, a statement about what the volume is not. The volume is, however, a sustained conversation between its contributors, a conversation that benefited greatly from sitting in the same room (and many restaurants) together over several days in Shanghai in early 2017, finding paths within and between our ideas. This assemble of historians, anthropologists, physicians and philosophers (most contributors have hyphens between these designations) took the global

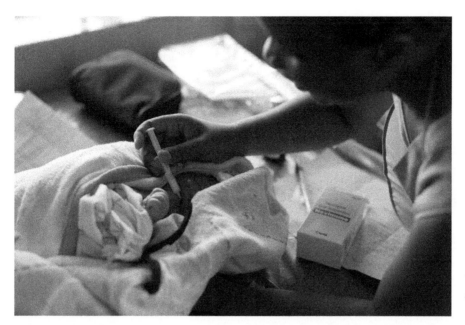

FIGURE 0.2: A newborn baby being given Nevimune; an antiviral medication to help prevent mother to baby transmission of HIV, Uganda, Africa. Credit: Mile 91/Ben Langdon / Alamy Stock Photo.

focus of our conversations back to North America, England and Western Europe, and then circled back through other geographies in the topics of their chapters. The result is a cultural history of medicine that, even while primarily attending to cases in 'the West', does so with an awareness and appreciation of the global implications of such a focus, including its limitations.

Chapter 1. In his chapter on 'Environment', Richard Keller examines the relationship between the environment and human health as a problem of both habitation and conceptualization. The chapter begins by looking at the way assumptions about human control of the environment (of cities, of the natural world) at the end of the nineteenth century led to twentieth-century anxieties about new ecological threats and the return of older problems. It is the perception of control and its loss in the face of a host of pressures – previously unseen disease vectors, changes in climate and environmental degradation, changing human and animal interactions – that organizes the chapter. HIV/AIDS and Lyme disease are the primary cases through which Keller weaves a story of a changing ecology of health and sickness, one framed and shaped by socio-political circumstances. The chapter concludes with more recent concerns about ecosystems and why shifts in transmissibility from vector-borne to sexual transmission of the Zika virus underscores perceived risks in the social environment.

What does it mean to control the environment? What would need to happen to make the reality of control (or even a sense of control) possible? Certainly the normalization and civic expectation of infrastructure at the end of the nineteenth century – from sanitation to cleaner air to safer living conditions to greater social order – sets the groundwork. But as Keller demonstrates, the thick confluence of environmental ruin, the production of social and biological conditions in which infectious disease flourish and hidden exposures (groundwater pollution or lead poisoning or violent crime or isolation [Keller, 2015]) steadily eroded these Gilded Age attitudes, not only reconfiguring the idea of what needed to be controlled, but fundamentally changing the notion of control itself. The various worlds in which humans found themselves became increasingly connected over the course of the twentieth century, but as sites of human habitation became more dense and unequal (and by extension animal habitats were encroached upon and thus uncomfortably shared with humans), control became a function of contact; zoonotic diseases jump between species and constricted environs produce new pressures. The 'environment' of human health is a vast domain, and as Keller shows in its many complementary and

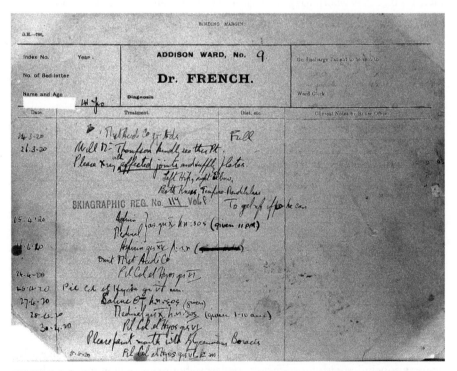

FIGURE 0.3: Dr. French, Addison Ward bed no. 9 (index no. 88), form for diagnosis, treatment etc., on blue paper, dated 29.3.1920- 5.5.1920; page 1. Credit: Wellcome Collection.

contributory forms, the social and the biological are bound together in unexpected and troubled ways. Keller demonstrates how crises foster environments of risks and thus new milieus of concern.

Chapter 2. In her chapter on 'Food', Nancy Chen examines how the interaction of the body and diet came to shape the definition of health during the twentieth century. When dietary standards and the regulation of food products were established, nutrients were placed into a biomedical framework. The line that had once separated food and medicine not only blurred, food became medicine. Chen explores the rise of nutraceuticals and other food products aimed at increasing longevity and improving human health. Patterns of food consumption (captured in the phrase 'you are what you eat') were not simply a means to a healthy lifestyle (or in the case of obesity, a pathway to morbidity), but were the primary mode by which a bodily ideal could be (and should be) achieved. In her chapter, Chen pulls together what would seem to be only loosely related threads – from food marketing and advertising, industrial food production, pharmaceutical development, campaigns of weight loss, new age remedies and traditional healing, and research on famine and malnutrition – to demonstrate how medicinal foodways or the configuring of food *as* medicine emerged as a powerful force of the culture of health in the twentieth century. The chapter offers a take on the topics in the chapters by Richard Keller and Robert Kirk through the discussion of microbial life and ingestion, fermentation, different ecologies (internal and external), epigenetics, diet and environmental exposures.

Chapter 3. In his chapter, 'Disease', Jeremy Greene outlines efforts to control disease and direct medical knowledge through classification and taxonomy. Greene traces how such efforts, even from the early moments of the century, reframed disease as *definable* and thus *controllable* – and as communicable diseases gave way to non-communicable, chronic conditions, the effort to identify and mitigate risk, as well as to intervene in the course of disease, created the conditions for a new system of therapeutics based on diagnostic assessment over communicated symptoms. Drawing on examples from his book *Prescribing by Numbers* (2008), Greene discusses how in the cases of diabetes and hypertension, treatment and prevention transformed most notably through the creation a new category of patienthood: the asymptomatic patient. Still, beyond the patient, 'knowing disease' through careful (though ever-evolving) classification advanced the notion that medicine was a science that could define disease as well as tame it.

A pivotal moment in the history the chapter explores is the transition that occurred mid-century, when the priorities of the medical and public health communities (and the resources offered by government and industry) to control and eradicate infectious disease were redirected toward chronic disease. As

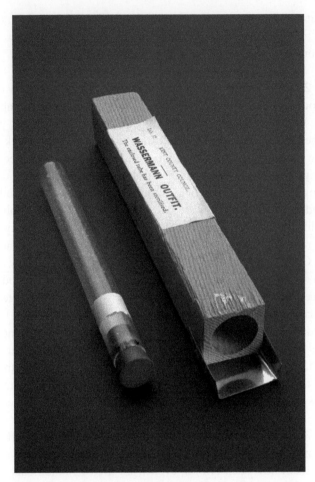

FIGURE 0.4: This glass bottle was used to take a blood sample and test for syphilis, a sexually transmitted infection. August von Wassermann (1866–1925), a German physician and bacteriologist, developed this diagnostic blood test in 1906. Shortly afterwards Paul Ehrlich and his team developed a cure for syphilis known as Salvarsan, the so-called 'magic bullet'. This required, however, a long period of treatment and was later replaced by the use of antibiotics such as penicillin. Credit: Science Museum, London.

Greene explains, 'lifestyle diseases' or 'diseases of civilization' (cancer, stroke, heart disease) in the United States and the United Kingdom overtook tuberculosis, pneumonia and diarrhoeal diseases as the leading causes of mortality. But how this transition was defined and represented says much about the way practitioners and researchers understood (and perhaps reimagined) their work. Nowhere do we see this effort more than in the nosological invention of new categories of disease and their measurement after this so-called epidemiological transition. No longer was the traffic in symptoms

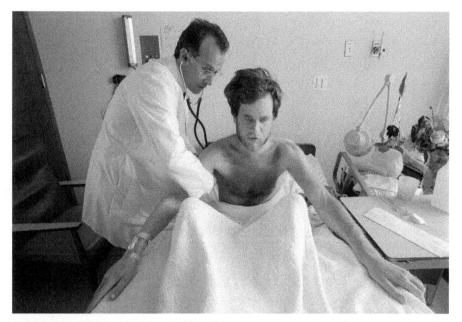

FIGURE 0.5: Physician Thomas J. Smith examines a man with AIDS at a Seattle hospital. Credit: Roger Ressmeyer / Corbis / VGG / Getty Images.

conveyed by patients or the subjective assessment through trained judgement of signs by practitioners during the clinical encounter central to treatment. Risk assessments, screenings technologies and the establishment of numerical thresholds all worked together to differentiate the normal from the pathological. The regulation of pharmaceutical manufacturing and the vast development of new drugs were responses to new markets of need around prevention and lifelong maintenance. This era of categorization in which diseases were put together and taken apart was still very much felt by patients, as standardization became the lens through which individuals were assessed and managed, and came to understand themselves.

Chapter 4. In his chapter, 'Animals', Robert Kirk opens with the curious story of Thomas Thwaites, the GoatMan, who attempted to close the gap between man and animal by living (for some time) as a goat. In the chapter, Kirk explores the relationship of humans and animals to one another and medicine's reliance on animals and animal models in the production of medical knowledge. By exploring the porous boundary between animal health and human health, as well as the entanglement of nature and culture, Kirk shows how medicine in the twentieth century has attempted to regulate this boundary in the control of disease. Much like Thwaites, Kirk makes a powerful intervention by blurring for a moment the

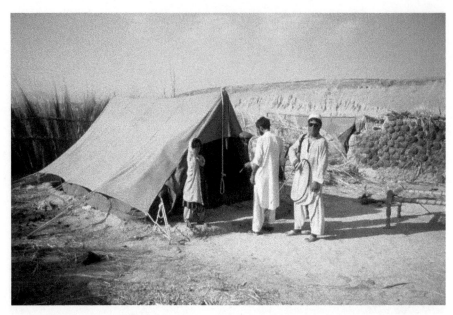

FIGURE 0.6: The inside of this tent in a refugee camp near Kabul, central Afghanistan is to be sprayed with residual insecticide. Note the mask and glasses protecting the sprayman's face. The refugee camp has been set up in an area endemic for cutaneous leishmaniasis due to *Leishmania tropica*. The vector *Phlebotomus sergenti* is highly anthropophilic, endophagic (feeding indoors) and endophilic. It is therefore possible to control this vector with residual spraying. Credit: Wellcome Collection/M Rowland.

line between human and animal, placing the 'nonhuman', 'post-human' and 'zoonotic' in the same field of vision in medical history and within the practice of medicine itself. The chapter forms a conceptual bridge between Richard Keller's chapter on 'Environment' through a discussion of the interaction of humans and animal/insect vectors and Nancy Chen's chapter on 'Food' through a discussion of industrialization in food production, here with a different set of actors and polemics. Kirk uses elaborate cases such as Creutzfeldt-Jakob disease and *kuru* in the highlands of Papua New Guinea – the former an animal precursor, bovine spongiform encephalopathy ('mad cow disease'), and the latter a related disease born of a cultural practice of endocannibalism (Lindenbaum, 1978) – to demonstrate the tight weave of animal health and human health (from food supply and biological semblance/transmissibility). Kirk shows how animals remain a vital resource for human medical (and physiological) knowledge throughout the century, and the debates that surround their use – from antivivisectionist discourse in the early century and to the necessity of nonhuman primates ('laboratory species') in medical research more recently.

Chapter 5. In his chapter on 'Objects', Cornelius Borck interrogates the conceptual taken-for-grantedness of first-aid kits, adhesive badges, dialysis

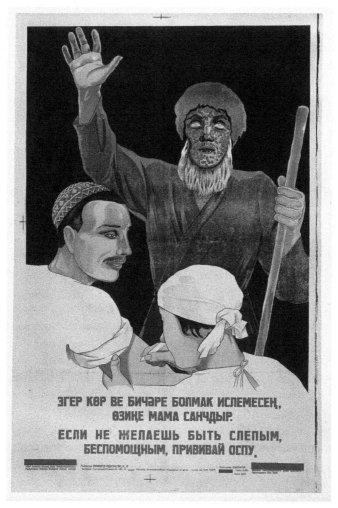

FIGURE 0.7: Vaccination against smallpox: a young Turkmen being vaccinated, contrasted with an elderly Turkmen who is blinded and disfigured by smallpox. Colour lithograph, between 1930 and 1939. Credit: Wellcome Collection.

machines, microscopes, CT scans and stethoscopes. The chapter considers the role of objects in biomedicine during the twentieth century, and emphasizes the significance of objects in the history of medicine despite their sketchy appearance in the telling of that history. Borck shows how objects play a decisive role in the medical encounter, shaping the terms of that encounter, and providing the means through which bodies and maladies are understood. The chapter is a philosophical intervention that reflects on the work medical objects have done to secure knowledge and represent the body and its internal processes. Instruments themselves are interventions, and their invention a window into the problems faced by practitioners and patients. But as Borck shows, medical instrumentation also paradoxically interferes with the practice of medicine, often increasing the objectification of patients and distancing the practitioner from them (the stethoscope being a buffer as much as an aid of contact and internal inspection), and sometimes depersonalizing them (the hospital gown). The symbolic capital held by these outwardly trivial yet vital apparatuses of medical knowledge and practice is formidable. In the chapter, Borck turns his attention to objects that are so domesticated within medicine they do not readily call out for notice. Yet these are not the afterthoughts of medical thinking and intervention, but a reflection of how medicine chooses to do its work, and how it understands (or misunderstands) that labour.

Chapter 6. In her chapter on 'Experience', public health historian and anthropologist Julie Livingston underlines the dimensions of human experience in biomedicine over the twentieth century by looking specifically at childbirth and death. The chapter considers how these principal life events are shaped and restyled along the lines of biomedical concern and intervention, exposing the transformative power of medicine on life and living. Livingston takes a conventional narrative of medical progress and puts it into conversation with otherwise minor voices of individuals and groups made vulnerable within the political economy of medical policies and practices. The result is a meditation on the concept of experience as one of an ongoing deliberation about the available terms for living and dying.

One key theme of this collection of essays, and at the centre of this chapter, is the supposition that in the twentieth century biomedicine enters the fold of human experience in novel and startling ways. In her chapter, Livingston peels back layers of this fold in order to explore the embodied, the political and the cultural dimensions of human illness and suffering. Her cases expose the reach of medicine *into* life, a reach that has the potential to prey on vulnerabilities as much as to alleviate suffering and prolong life. It will not surprise readers to learn that medicine has political dimensions. Even the clinical encounter, if always already a contest between healer and the sick, became intensified along political and highly personal lines over the past century. As Livingston shows, the terms that medical ideology takes on (in the case of eugenics, for instance) bores deeply into public and private life, creating an intimacy between medicine and life, and thus changing the terms of civic life (in the case of activism centred around disability or sexuality, for instance) in ways that blend the biological and the political.

Livingston uses powerful examples from childbirth and dying, pregnancy and motherhood, and toxic exposure and recuperation to show how medicine has come to change the terms of life and living. Life (its possibility, the events that define it) is increasing mediated by medical technologies and sites of medical offering (the move from home births to the hospital births, or in the other direction from the hospital to the hospice, for example), thus generating a different (and evolving) set of expectations and norms. But *experience* in Livingston's chapter is not restricted to that which is felt *within* the body (and how medicine chooses to regard that inner experience or feltness): experience is a concept the reworks medicine's relationship to humans across the lifespan, offering a different weave of risks, rights, privileges, affordances and deficiencies. Perhaps most significantly, in the chapter Livingston demonstrates that even a concept as seemingly universal as human experience is itself fundamentally uneven and unequal in its expressions.

Chapter 7. In his chapter, 'Mind and Brain', Rhodri Hayward begins by declaring: 'The mind and brain sciences make their own histories, although these are histories that most academic historians would struggle to recognize.' In part, the making of the histories of the mind and brain sciences can be found in the contours formed by the public (as much as the professional, though perhaps more so) attention given to it, including providing its record or archive. These histories, shared between the branches of medicine under the header 'mind and brain sciences', are the means through which various actors express their own self-understanding and demonstrate self-awareness.

In the chapter, Hayward outlines the transformation of nineteenth-century psychiatry and neurology into a basis for the modern neurosciences, and considers the implications of this transformation, and of the mind and brain sciences securing a (perhaps *the*) principal place in medical thinking in the twentieth century. Hayward shows how therapeutic promise and the potential to predict and guide human behaviours fomented a reorientation of psychological medicine and reformed its institutions. The chapter shows in great detail how, within the brain sciences, we find the same modes and tendencies of standardization, categorization, screening and diagnosis, and therapeutic offering (ultimately in the form of psychopharmaceutical intervention for the amelioration of suffering) described in Greene's chapter, thus marking a more general (and potent) shift in medicine thinking and practice, somehow beyond the brain.

Chapter 8. In this final chapter on 'Authority', George Weisz asks us to pause for a moment to consider what we mean by the phrase 'medical authority' – a phrase that seems to have so much currency in debates about what is wrong and perhaps dangerous about medicine today. In this phrase, are we acknowledging the power of the individual physician, or a group of professional elites, or even a body of credible knowledge, or something altogether different? In order to get to the heart of the concept of authority within the medical profession, Weisz first examines the ways physicians are challenged both in the marketplace and through the scrutiny of their decision-making. The chapter then moves to the concept of medical authority related not to individual practitioners but to groups of professionals who became increasingly organized and who find ways to regulate themselves over the course of the twentieth century. Weisz traces the rise of standardization in medical education and training, and the creation of systems of certification and licensing by physicians and other stakeholders. The chapter further explores the management of practitioners, the diffusion of oversight and clinical decision-making across an array of administrators and other health professionals, and the role and management of medical error.

In the stream of standardization, institutional establishment and technological expertise, 'authority' became medicine's watchword in the twentieth century. But as Weisz shows, there are diffuse expressions to this authority and a disparate set of actors who hold and exercise it. The role that health administrators and other health professionals played in creating systems of education, oversight, discipline and regulation of medical practitioners should not be overlooked (though they often are) in the establishment of medicine as authoritative. Weisz reflects on how different forms of self-regulation by physicians, various licensing and medical stakeholders, the establishment of professional rules, norms of practice, management of practitioners and the rise of elite medical schools fed a societal ideal of control held by those in the profession, while simultaneously exposing various means of authority and control to which practitioners were themselves beholden.

The history of medicine always seems to be closing and reopening, or perhaps it is simply fixed in the continuous present where its priorities are rethought and retested – an existential problem of the here and now (Hayward, 2005). In this volume, the contributors have sought to present critical perspectives on a cultural history of medicine in the twentieth century in a manner that invites further thought and examination. Because the cases remain so close to our present moment, it is nearly impossible not to think of them in current terms. Said another way, these essays were written before Covid-19 was part of our lexicon, and were published after we were forced to rethink our relationships with healthcare, medicine, and each other. With this in mind, the volume is neither a primer nor a final word; it is a guide for what might be ways to think through the impact and reach of medicine over the past century, a reach both veiled and apparent, and one that extends into today, whatever today might hold.

CHAPTER ONE

Environment

RICHARD C. KELLER

At the turn of the twentieth century, the environment was an entity to be conquered, tamed and managed through human ingenuity. The rapid urbanization of the nineteenth century created a need for dramatic city planning projects that generated the modern urban environment. In London, Paris, Vienna, New York, Chicago and beyond, subterranean networks of sanitation mirrored the surface landscapes of habitability, providing clean water to the city while sluicing toxic effluent away. Cities became machines for living, technological interventions that endlessly battled the entropy of the restless nature that threatened buildings with decay, streets with weather and bodies with disease. Investment in urban infrastructure – combined with developments in vaccination, food preservation, water filtration and agricultural production – indicated that a tamed environment was a healthy environment, which data about health and life expectancy appeared to support in the first decades of the twentieth century.

By the end of the twentieth century, this rosy view of the taming of nature had largely eroded. Where the shackling of nature in the service of human interest was a narrative of progress in the past, it became a dystopian one at the millennium. Mass extinctions, a menacing climate crisis, irreversible pollution, plastics that are incapable of degradation – all with anthropogenic origins – have replaced the notion of an orderly dominion over nature as the principal sign of humanity's place in the landscape. People have shifted the world out of balance, with measurably permanent effects on the health of populations and their environments.

This chapter discusses global health and the environment in the past century by exploring changing anthropogenic threats to human health. It does so by examining the relationship between body and environment in three particular frames: those of infectious disease (with attention to plague, HIV/AIDS and Lyme disease), cancer, and the notion of the body as an environment in its own right. It figures the environment in the broad sense of human surroundings, and examines the ways in which medical, epidemiological and hygienic thinking have engaged this concept in the past hundred years. For reasons of space and coherence, this chapter leaves a great deal out of the story: it spends little time on the built environment, it contains very little discussion of occupational health and it avoids discussion of natural and human-made disasters. This is not because these aspects are unimportant to the narrative of environment and health: they are critical and richly developed areas of the field (Murphy, 2006; Rosner and Markowitz, 2006; Steinberg, 2001). Rather, this chapter presents a story about disease and the environment that seeks to develop a notion of the anthropogenic body and the conditions of its making, its vulnerability and its exposure to hazards by focusing on a limited number of cases.

The ecology of sickness and health has evolved dramatically over the course of the past hundred years, from paradigms organized primarily by germ theories of disease now becoming complicated by social-ecological models that account for broad intersections of human, animal and environmental health. In an era that many consider to be the 'Anthropocene', or an epoch in which people have become the defining force that shapes the Earth's environment, the notion of a human determinism of sickness and health – people, rather than climates, are the true environment of disease – is tempting to consider. But it is also important to recognize that people's interactions with their environments – and therefore their exposures and vulnerabilities to environmental hazards – have differed dramatically over the course of the past century.

HEALTH AND DISEASE IN AN ECOLOGICAL FRAME

The environment is perhaps best conceptualized not as nature or wilderness, but instead as a series of relations between human and exterior worlds. As the environmental historian Linda Nash has argued, people are enmeshed in human, artificial and natural systems (Nash, 2006). The environment constitutes the forms of nature that exist outside of human intervention, but also the places that humans have shaped around them. And no environment is free of hazards. Hazards to health are potential environmental threats, which assume meaning when combined with exposure and vulnerability. Hazards that are inherent to human surroundings include disasters such as earthquakes and floods, but also groundwater pollution, lead poisoning, and violent crime. As John Higginson, Director of the World Health Organization's International Agency for Research on Cancer, argued in 1979, the environment is 'cultural as well as chemical', including 'the air you breathe, the culture you live in, the agricultural habits of your community, the social cultural habits, the social pressures, the physical chemicals with which you come into contact, the diet and so on' (Maugh, 1978).

The environment thus constitutes a milieu in which we circulate and which shapes our experience – one that can be either conducive or hazardous to health. Vulnerable populations are those who not only are subject to inordinate environmental hazards, but also have limited shelter from those hazards and a limited ability to respond to them. Environmental health risk, then, develops as a function of a proximate hazard, the extent of exposure, its potential consequences and an inability to avoid or resist that hazard (Comfort, 1999).

Questions about environmental risk and its implications for sickness and health are ancient. In the Western tradition, they date at least to Hippocrates, who in *Airs, Waters, Places* posits health as a function of equilibrium between the body and its surroundings. By the early modern period, medical geography was an entrenched specialization that sought to merge understandings about climate and constitution with the global mission of an expanding Europe. But the importance of 'environment' for sickness and health went far beyond climate and latitude. By the early nineteenth century, rapid urbanization in Europe and the United States facilitated the emergence of a new sort of medical geography, one that focused on the social disparities of sickness and health that characterized growing cities. Social reformers such as Edwin Chadwick described horrific living conditions among English workers as a function of their immorality and the failings of the English poor laws, while Friedrich Engels, exploring some of the same burgeoning industrial cities, saw these conditions as inherent qualities of capitalism, in which an economic geography of class predisposed vulnerable English workers to poor health outcomes due to pollution and disease. On the continent, the physician and economist Louis-René Villermé mapped an economic geography of life and death in Paris that ultimately led to the reconstruction of the city, largely on hygienist grounds.

By the late nineteenth century, a radical turn began to decentre environmental approaches to public health. The emergence of bacteriology, beginning in the 1860s, allowed for a new framing of disease in narrower terms. The notion that environments on a grand scale shaped sickness and health gradually gave way to the idea that particular agents were primarily responsible for the disease burden. Cholera or tuberculosis were less a function of a noisome stench of poverty, and were more closely linked to microbes that followed predictable patterns of transmission. The total yielded to the specific. To be sure, there remained important environmental components to infectious disease transmission. Yet it is clear that the embracing of a bacteriological (and later virological) model of disease pushed public health policy away from broadly environmental approaches towards what scientists and health policymakers saw as the choke point of disease: the highly specific pathways of infection.

INFECTIOUS ECOLOGIES

Bacteriology and changing concepts of environment: plague

Although bacteriological approaches scaled down public health policy to the level of the microbe, ecological concerns remained critical to understanding the propagation of disease in specific contexts. Bacteriology's rise did not so much mean that the environment no longer mattered: instead, the discipline forced a reconceptualization of what constituted the relevant environment for disease. The third plague pandemic, which began near the end of the nineteenth century and stretched to the mid-twentieth century, offers a useful example. The medical historian Andrew Cunningham argues that the third pandemic crystallized the emerging discipline of bacteriology by confirming the place of the laboratory in the diagnosis of disease: although clinical assessments remained important, the definitive identification of a pathogen in a laboratory setting became the *sine qua non* of disease. In this ontological framing of illness, the microbe effectively became the disease (Cunningham, 1992).

While there is some truth to this conceptualization, environmental factors remained central to the understanding of plague and its transmission. Reducing the disease to its pathogen disallowed for a broader understanding of how a given disease could flourish in one environment and perish in another. It failed to distinguish between the agent of disease and the processes of propagation and infection. Colonial administrators in India, China, Hong Kong and South Africa remained convinced that poverty, the intermingling of human and animal spaces, and filth were critical determinants of risk for plague transmission (Simpson, 1905). A broader environmental reading enabled the explanation of critical disparities in the pandemic, such as an unequal mortality burden in which more than 180,000 died of plague in Bombay, while only about 500 died in San Francisco (Echenberg, 2002, 2017; Swanson, 1977; Craddock, 2000).

The work of the nascent Pasteur Institutes on plague underscored the importance of environmental factors as important facilitators of microbial transmission. Working in Hong Kong and Indochina, Alexandre Yersin studied the plague bacillus intently under the microscope, but also in a range of other settings. The careful notation of symptoms, the identification of an agent, the recreation of a model epidemic and the effort to develop working sera or immunizations took place in the laboratory and the clinic, but such efforts were doomed to fail in the absence of a careful mapping of the geography of disease, an understanding of interspecies contact, a careful examination of urban layout and interactions, and a keen awareness of population behaviour: the ecological factors that shaped exposure and vulnerability to a disease hazard. The *Annales de l'Institut Pasteur*, the journal of the global network of Pasteur Institutes, teems with studies that plotted plague case incidence alongside factors such as rat mortality, rainfall, temperature, neighbourhood composition and ethnicity in an effort to understand the working of disease in urban space (Latour, 1988). Such work led to the Pasteurian Paul-Louis Simond's documentation of a rat-flea-human nexus critical to the transmission of plague, along with the eventual understanding of plague as primarily a disease of rodents that only occasionally jumped into human populations through flea vectors. In a pre-antibiotic era, the leading approach to plague control then became intense raticide programmes, with public health agencies deploying poison and employing people and dogs to kill rats in American, European and colonial cities (Vann, 2003).

Sporadic outbreaks of plague in global port cities marked the pandemic through the mid-twentieth century, including Oran, Tunis, Cape Town, Porto, Dakar, Port-Saïd, Lima and Antananarivo (Echenberg, 2007). Yet the epidemic in Manchuria in 1910 and 1911 stands out for its virulence as well as its eventual contribution to the imagining of disease in an ecological frame. In contrast to other regions, Manchuria experienced pneumonic rather than strictly bubonic plague, meaning the disease was transferred from person to person as well as through flea vectors. The epidemic also exploited an ecology of economic development and labour migration as consequences of the Boxer Rebellion and the Russo-Japanese War. The region was desolate as a result of the war, prompting significant Japanese investment in new ports and rail lines. This development coincided with a dramatic increase in the demand for the furs of Manchuria's plentiful marmots, as innovations in chemical dyes allowed their inferior furs to mimic the far more expensive furs of sable or mink. Farmers suffering from the economic dislocation prompted by the Boxer Rebellion migrated to Manchuria on these new transportation networks, where hunting marmots – which were a principal reservoir for sylvatic plague in the region – proved far more lucrative than farming. Knowing the dangers of weak

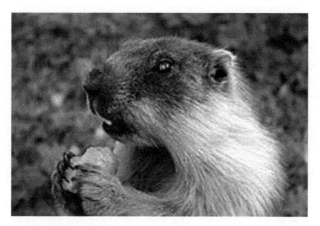

FIGURE 1.1: The Tarbagan Marmot: a reservoir of plague in China and Siberia. Credit: Wikimedia Commons.

or dead animals, locals had long avoided them and suffered relatively few cases of plague. The newcomers were less careful, often taking the furs of sick and dead marmots that were easier to harvest. Likely as a function of this breach of protocols, plague exploded among the migrant population and spread quickly when a pneumonic strain emerged. The plague killed between 45,000 and 60,000 in just a few months, with health workers unable to bury the bodies once a brutal winter froze the ground (McNeill, 1976; Jones, 2011; Summers, 2012).

Although clearly linked to bacterial infection, plague thus exploits particular ecologies to erupt in human populations. It relies on specific political economies such as the aftermath of war and economic migration in Manchuria, colonial trade networks in port cities, patterns of urban segregation and interspecies contact. The presence of the microbe does not equal the making of an epidemic: the disease is widespread among prairie dogs in the American Southwest, for example, but only results in a handful of human cases every year. Rather, it is a particular set of environmental circumstances – and the place of often vulnerable human populations within that geography – that comprise exposure and risk.

Changing human geographies and ecologies: HIV/AIDS

Plague is a rodent disease that affects humans in the right circumstances. It is like a number of other zoonotic diseases, such as hantaviruses and avian influenza virus, which can be devastating in humans, but which are primarily infections that prey on their animal hosts. Simian immunodeficiency virus (SIV) differs from these other zoonotic diseases. It only rarely causes serious disease in nonhuman primates, but its human equivalent causes staggering mortality. Like the other examples, however, HIV relies on highly specific ecologies to reach peak lethality. Both in its original emergence and spread in West and Central Africa in the early twentieth century and its explosion in the United States and Western Europe in the 1980s, SIV/HIV took advantage of changing ecologies to generate important epidemiological change. Transformations in the couplings of humans and nature as well as an altered social milieu generated new vulnerabilities that fell prey to an opportunistic hazard.

Since at least the late 1980s, biomedical researchers have looked to Central and West Africa as the crucible of HIV/AIDS. Primatologists and virologists have combed rainforests in search of evidence of the species jump. By comparing traces of shed virus in a range of nonhuman primates, they have estimated that the two different types of HIV migrated from simians to humans in multiple transmissions between the 1910s and the 1950s (Essex and Kanki, 1988; Hahn and Shaw, 2000; Sharp and Hahn, 2011). Biomedical scientists have built on this hypothesis to develop historical theories about the factors that drove SIV into human populations. They have extrapolated from a widely accepted fact – the species jump, most likely from chimpanzees, in this forty-year period – to construct possible historical re-enactments of the environmental transformation of an entire region and its dire epidemiological consequences.

The core of most of these narratives is the 'cut hunter' theory (Wolfe et al., 2005; Weiss and Wrangham, 1999). According to this hypothesis, hunting and butchering of chimpanzees led to the introduction of simian blood into humans, providing a mechanism for the transfer of the virus. Although hominins have hunted other primates for millions of years, virologists have argued that colonial transformations of the political economy of labour and sexuality are to blame for this spillover (Pepin, 2011). The harvesting of wild rubber constructed new patterns of labour migration and hunting that increased the likelihood of cross-species transmission. The development of colonial railways and road networks facilitated processes of urbanization and new patterns of sexuality and sex work that were favourable to the virus's propagation in the Congo and eventually beyond (Freed, 2010). Research drawing on population genetics and viral sequencing supported these claims, documenting plausible patterns of the virus's spread through these colonial transportation networks from city to city and village to village (Faria et al., 2014).

These works often drew conclusions based on crude assumptions about caricatures of colonial society as an exclusive agent of change in central Africa. They frequently ignored well-documented histories of urbanization and migration that long preceded the colonial period, and their modelling of sexual transmission extrapolates from contemporary transmission patterns and assume these would apply to the past as well. Yet despite the lack of historical nuance, circumstantial evidence suggests that, as Tamara Giles-Vernick has argued, 'specific historical and local ecologies – including medical technologies, patterns of gender and sexual relations, as well as broader structural factors – primarily shaped the geography and temporality of the HIV epidemic' (Giles-Vernick et al., 2013). Ecological changes in this period – including perhaps new hunting strategies and practices, intensified migration and new gender relations, among other transformations – were critical to the exacerbation of the hazard of a simian virus that could infect humans in central Africa, provoking new or more intense exposures with the capacity to prey on developing vulnerabilities.

Such transformations were also critical to the spread of HIV/AIDS in the United States and Western Europe, where the epidemic took advantage of decades of social change that preceded the 1980s. The burgeoning epidemic in the global North relied on new forms of social interaction and transformations of urban space and politics in the post-war era, including changing attitudes to sexuality, rising incidence of drug use and addiction, and new medical technological developments that transformed markets for blood and blood products.

The notion of wholesome 1950s conformity with young couples saving their sexuality for marriage was always more a white middle-class caricature than a reality, but several factors transformed sexuality beginning in the early 1960s. The advent of the contraceptive pill provided women who could access it the ability to take control of their sexuality and freed them from the biological burden of pregnancy (while social pressures continued to hold women to a sexual double standard). Changing social mores allowed sex for heterosexual and same-sex couples alike to become a venue for political expression, an opportunity to reject the conformism of the 1950s and the pre-war era (Watkins, 2016). The emergence of safe havens for gays and lesbians in some American cities in the 1970s consequently altered the sexual ecology of those urban spaces, as did the effectiveness of antibiotics such as penicillin, which helped foster a broad complacency about sexually transmitted infections.

A loosening of American attitudes towards sexuality (along with similar developments in Europe) brought moral outrage to a fever pitch with the beginnings of the AIDS epidemic. Figures on the Christian Right denounced the free love movement and homosexual behaviour as the culprit for a new sexually transmitted disease: 'immoral' sexual 'deviants' were reaping what they had sown. This extended to some within the gay community. The San Francisco journalist Randy Shilts famously condemned what he called the promiscuity of gay men in the city, with lurid descriptions of anonymous encounters in San Francisco's bathhouses and tales of gay men who had hundreds if not thousands of partners in any given year, while New York gay activist Larry Kramer had written presciently in 1978, 'it all needs to change … before you fuck yourself to death' (Shilts, 1987; Bersani, 1995, 2009; Brandt, 1988; Treichler, 1999).

These responses contain the hyperbole typical of the period's culture wars, exacerbated by an atmosphere of crisis and uncertainty. They also embodied the homophobia inherent to a medical profession that had long considered homosexuality not only deviant but also pathological. But despite the moralizing excess of reactionaries, the period did witness a significant increase in the reporting of sexually transmitted diseases. Reported cases of syphilis quadrupled between 1965 and 1975, gonorrhoea surpassed chicken pox as the leading infectious disease in the United States and the rise of Herpes Simplex II in the late 1970s served as a warning sign of emerging diseases linked to sex with concurrent partners (Garrett, 1995). Moreover, widespread STIs often produced lesions that created a direct pathway for viruses such as HIV to enter the bloodstream.

A second critical ecological transformation concerned America's cities. Where some city centres thrived in the post-war period, many witnessed significant decline as a paradoxical function of economic development. As the post-war boom drew many of the wealthiest urbanites to flee to the suburbs, many cities faced dramatic losses of tax revenue, with powerful effects on schools, public spaces and city services. Other developments exacerbated this effect. Cheaper land and interstate highway exchanges that bypassed cities altogether created incentives for major employers to abandon urban spaces and relocate to exurban sites. As factories left the cities, so too did stable employment. Even flourishing cities witnessed neighbourhood-specific decline, with examples including Chicago's south side, the Bronx and Harlem in New York, and south-central Los Angeles. Broad economic decline left the informal economy as a principal survival mechanism for many trapped in a cycle of underemployment and under-education (Cohen, 1999; Bourgois, 1995). The arrival of the Vietnam War and inequalities of a conscription burden that bore more heavily on blacks than whites and on the poor than on the middle class aggravated the problems of the city. Easy access to heroin in Vietnam left many addicted, while cycling through tours of duty facilitated the importation of South-East Asian heroin in to the United States. Self-reported addiction rates skyrocketed in the US, with the greatest concentration in cities (Robins et al., 2010).

Panic about marijuana use among whites in the suburbs combined with a fear of heroin addiction prompted President Nixon to declare the War on Drugs in 1971. The administration saw multiple political benefits in this action: by tapping into fears of drugs, the criminalization of drug use broke apart the anti-war movement and urban black communities (Baum, 2016). Yet one unforeseen consequence exacerbated the harms of drug injection. The criminalization of paraphernalia drove drug injection underground. To avoid carrying syringes, cookers or other paraphernalia that could lead to arrest, users could pay to use equipment provided by an underground shooting gallery. This created an economic incentive for the intensified reuse and sharing of needles (Bourgois, 1998).

As the anthropologist Philippe Bourgois has illustrated through extensive fieldwork, social hierarchies among homeless injecting drug users also fuel risky behaviour. Those who are able to earn regular income through employment, panhandling, theft or other means are more easily able to maintain regular injection habits and are the least likely to be forced to share drugs, syringes or other equipment. By contrast, those with the least earning power are forced to rely on the charity of those around them in order to maintain their habits, and often resort to using leftover syringes and used cotton filters, extracting what they are able in order to stave off withdrawal. Such activities naturally increase their exposure to HIV and other pathogens, intensifying the cycle of sickness, dependency and vulnerability (Bourgois et al., 1997; Bourgois, 2009).

Just as Pepin and others are perhaps too casual in referring to phenomena such as urbanization, migration and changing sexual practices as the precondition of an African AIDS epidemic, there are dangers in drawing on vaguely defined sexual liberation and urban decline as the root cause of an epidemic in the global North. There are other critical developments to consider. The role of sexual tourism in spreading the disease – particularly in Latin America and the Caribbean, as well as in South-East Asia – remains under-examined by historians. Blood transfusion was also central to the spread of HIV in the United States. The formation of a national network of blood banks in 1947, the rapid expansion of blood banking after the invention of the plastic blood bag in 1948 and the development of powerful new clotting agents in 1965 all contributed to the proliferation of blood and plasma donation, collection, sales and distribution (Lederer, 2008). While the sale of plasma as an economic survival strategy for drug users has long been well known, less attention has been paid to the practice among gay men in an era of rampant employment and housing discrimination against homosexuals. The desperation of the addict is a regular trope in this literature. The notion of the gay man as well-educated and easily dissuaded from donating blood or selling plasma is every bit as much a stereotype, and one worthy of close examination. But it remains clear that changing sexual environments, patterns of drug use and biomedical technologies all contributed to an ecology that proved favourable to an emerging virus, provoking broad exposure to a new hazard among vulnerable populations.

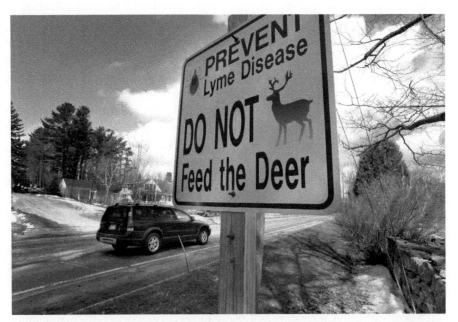

FIGURE 1.2: New suburban neighbourhoods generated an ideal environment for the emergence of Lyme disease in the United States. In 2011 Cumberland erected signs warning people about feeding deer, which can transmit lime disease. Credit: Portland Press Herald / Contributor / Getty Images.

First-world problems: Lyme disease in America

The Second World War had pulled Americans out of the Great Depression by offering full employment, but shortages and rationing left them with little to purchase with their savings. The post-war era brought with it a spending boom, and programmes such as the GI Bill and highway construction combined with a new consumer ethos (as well as earlier interventions such as the home mortgage interest deduction) to offer many Americans the dream of home ownership in the suburbs. Neighbourhoods dotted with small ranch houses that could easily be expanded on large lots exploded in the counties surrounding American cities, providing affordable housing for those who could leave the city and its attendant pathologies behind (Rome, 2001). A myth of suburban salubrity became the backdrop of aspirational America, while the age-old notion of the city as a site of pathology acquired new meaning as middle-class whites increasingly left the city behind (Mitman, 2005; Rosenberg, 1998; Milgram, 1970; Walkowitz, 1992).

Suburban sprawl in post-war America did not merely deprive many cities of their tax base. One of the profound ironies of suburban development is that a move intended to allow people to raise their families in a healthier alternative to the city generated a range of new pathologies. The rise of the automobile-dependent city has introduced an array of new risks. More driving has increased air pollution as well as accident risk, and has encouraged more sedentary lifestyles. Auto accidents are a leading cause of injury and death in the United States, with exposure to this hazard increasing with every new suburban development that requires automotive transport for access. Respiratory disease as a function of particulate pollution, but also as a function of allergy and mould-exposure linked to new building techniques, has proliferated. Rising rates of obesity and depression have followed the expansion of a sedentary lifestyle and the relative isolation of suburban life.

Among the most significant health risks that evolved with expanding suburbs are those associated with land-cover change. Low-density development usually requires the transformation of landscapes, initiating new wildland-urban interfaces. Beginning in the mid-1970s, the insatiable appetite for suburban conquest that began in the immediate post-war period had yielded a frightening new illness phenomenon. A cluster of cases of juvenile rheumatoid arthritis appeared in Lyme and Old Lyme, Connecticut, which lent their names to the disease. The disease itself was not new: settlers in New England had described a similar illness characterized by joint pain, fevers and a circular rash centuries earlier, and observers in Europe had even identified the tick as connected with the disease well before the vector concept had developed. But the epidemic nature of the disease was new, with a proliferation of cases in the 1970s, 1980s and 1990s, as well as a spread of those cases outside of New England to the Middle Atlantic States and the Upper Midwest (Edlow, 2003).

The disease's expansion uniformly followed increasing suburban and exurban development (Cromley et al., 1998). It relied on a complex tangle of processes that transformed local environments and created new opportunities for exposure to this hazard. Sprawl in New England followed a multilayered process of land-use change. Beginning in the seventeenth century, settlers cut down old growth forests to construct farms. The decline of New England agriculture in the late nineteenth and early twentieth centuries led to the abandonment of these farms, when they were taken over by secondary-growth forest and a renewal of local biodiversity (Barbour, 2015). Post-war suburbanization again targeted these forests, this time fragmenting them rather than levelling them wholesale. New wooded developments provided green spaces surrounded by 'nature' for those who could afford them. They offered a haven from the city for the commuter, who could travel from a suburb in Connecticut, Rhode Island or Massachusetts into any of a number of cities for work, while avoiding the city's high taxes, pollution and crime. Children could attend homogeneous schools that were unofficially segregated as a function of economic inequality, and spend their afternoons and weekends playing in the healthy spaces of the woods and on their lush green lawns and gardens.

But such developments also devastated the biodiversity of these regions. Predators found the environment unwelcome and either died or migrated elsewhere. As a result, deer and certain species of mice proliferated while others declined (Patz et al., 2004; Patz, et al., 2008). Meanwhile, easy access to this manufactured nature also generated new forms of interspecies contact. Suburban gardens offered plentiful food sources for deer and white-footed mice, effective carriers of deer ticks and Lyme bacteria, respectively. The ticks that were a nuisance of summers spent in the woods and on green lawns – that were carried into the house by the family dog or cat – became by the 1970s the carriers of a chronic disease that became a scourge of middle-class America.

As a pathology of privilege, Lyme disease also transformed the milieu of the doctor-patient encounter, with effects for a clinical environment organized around physician expertise and the dispensing of care. While physicians saw Lyme disease as a bacterial infection that responded to antibiotic treatment (if caught in time), patients often experienced chronic sequelae of what they saw as a protean entity that proved elusive to treatment (Aronowitz, 2012). As a function of the relative affluence of many of those initially afflicted by the disease, patient advocacy groups emerged relatively quickly, often supported by sympathetic physicians (known as 'Lyme literate' among advocates). This phenomenon upset medical consensus on the disease, leading to prolonged battles over the development of treatments and vaccines, often fought on epistemological grounds: where a vaccine might prove effective in preventing infections, it also had the capacity to threaten the identity of the chronic Lyme patient by invalidating the illness experience.

CHRONIC DISEASE: CANCER IN AN EVOLVING LANDSCAPE OF RISK

Although infectious disease occupies the most prominent place in the global health agenda, non-communicable diseases (NCDs) have emerged as fast-growing risks on a global scale. The health transition model that curried favour in the epidemiological community in the 1960s and 1970s proposed that economic development would lessen the burden of infectious disease in industrialized countries, which would experience higher levels of chronic diseases such as heart disease, cancer and diabetes. Infectious disease would remain the province of developing countries, which had low rates of vaccination, poor sanitation infrastructure and pervasive unclean water.

Yet by the turn of the twenty-first century, this model has proven woefully inadequate. Economic inequality and ecological change have contributed to emerging and resurgent infectious diseases in the global North, shattering the complacency of the mid-twentieth century. Meanwhile, although much of the developing world struggles profoundly against a disproportionate infectious disease burden, surging rates of NCDs have opened a new battlefront in the countries least able to cope with this new challenge. Moreover, much of the NCD burden is closely linked to environmental and social factors such as changing exposures, diets and behaviours in both the global North and South.

Carcinogens such as arsenic, uranium and ultraviolet radiation have always existed in human surroundings. Likewise, random genetic mutations have probably always caused rare cancers in humans. Yet many have considered cancer the anthropogenic disease par excellence, with some calling it a 'disease of civilization' (Stefansson, 1960; Proctor, 1995; Maugh, 1978). Patients, physicians and scientists have long recognized the connection between industrialization and rising cancer rates, with a specific emphasis on chemical exposure as an occupational hazard. Until the early twentieth century, these were mostly correlations: a British physician noted extensive cancer rates among chimney sweeps in the late eighteenth century, speculating that soot exposure was the cause, while exposure to tar and coal smoke correlated closely with rising cancer incidence throughout Europe a century later (Carson, 2002). German scientists documented connections between uranium mining and lung cancer in the 1870s, and between dye manufacture and bladder cancer in 1895 (Proctor, 1999). Within a few decades, scientists began to demonstrate causality by recreating these cancers in the laboratory: in France, Germany, Japan, England and the United States important connections were revealed between chemical or radiation exposure and cancer in animals, while every year brought new correlations to public attention (Proctor, 1995).

Cancer appeared to be on track to supersede infectious diseases as the principal public health threat of the twentieth century in industrialized countries. Yet there was significant debate about whether the disease itself was increasing, or if there was merely an increase in diagnosis. Both are likely true. Although diagnoses were increasing rapidly with new histological methods that provided specific insights into neoplastic growth, environmental exposure to carcinogens – through both occupation and lifestyle – were increasing even more dramatically. Industrialization and urbanization brought with them significant increases in exposure to pollutants, while high rates of tobacco and alcohol consumption also played critical roles in rising cancer prevalence.

Surging rates of cancer in the twentieth century also pointed to a central paradox in the notion of cancer as a disease of civilization. When Europeans and Americans referred to cancer as a sort of index of development in the nineteenth century, they often considered it to be the price of living in a society marked by material progress. By the mid-twentieth century, the health transitions model suggested much the same: infectious disease faded and cancer rates rose as a function of economic development. For some, this was also an indication of increasing moral weakness: as the historian Robert Proctor has argued, much of the Nazi war on cancer inveighed against insidious habits such as smoking, alcohol consumption and a sedentary lifestyle (Proctor, 1999; Proctor, 2012).

But there is an important paradox in this notion as well. Although many saw cancer as a disease of development, cancer has historically preyed on the subaltern populations that have faced the greatest exposure to environmental toxins. Critical examples of vulnerable populations include small children who swept chimneys, women workers who painted luminous numbers on wristwatch dials with radium paint, Navajo uranium miners in the United States, soldiers who handled defoliants such as Agent Orange and the rural Vietnamese populations on whom it rained, and agricultural labourers who face near-constant exposure to pesticides (Moore, 2016; Pasternak, 2011; Reagan, 2011). Moreover, the chronic burden of diseases such as cancer exacerbates poverty. Disease-related disability often entails the loss of employment, while expensive treatments strain resources. Worse still, in areas where environmental exposure has produced cancer clusters – examples include Hinkley (California), Toms River (New Jersey) and Woburn (Massachusetts) – victims' houses become unsellable, leading many to bankruptcy.

Meanwhile, exploding cancer rates in developing countries are now casting doubt on the notion that cancer was ever purely a disease linked to material progress. The *Global Burden of Disease* update published in 2008 notes that NCDs including cancer cause a fifth of all deaths in sub-Saharan Africa, half of all deaths in South and South-East Asia, two-thirds of all deaths in Latin America and three-quarters of all deaths in East Asia. Cancer in particular is the second-leading cause of death in the developing world, killing more than 5 million in developing countries in 2004 alone (World Health Organization, 2008). The rate is highest in low-middle income countries, where disposable income allows for high rates of tobacco and alcohol consumption, and where resources for education and the struggle against cancer are few (Livingston, 2012).

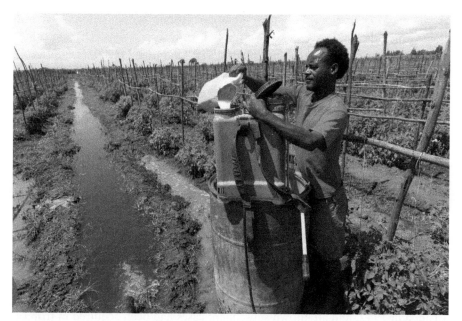

FIGURE 1.3: At least since the 1960s, scientists have linked exposure to pesticides and other toxins to cancer. Low-wage agricultural workers and factory labourers, as well as poor communities in which waste dumps have been sited, face the highest levels of exposure. Meki River delta, Ziway, Ethiopia, October 2013. A day labourer on this irrigated tomato plantation is filling his backpack to spray insecticide, Credit: Mike Goldwater / Alamy Stock Photo.

Rather than a disease of 'civilization', cancer is a disease of exposure and vulnerability. Economic development yields capital, but also profound inequality. While some gain significant resources, many more gain exposure to the hazards of development. This phenomenon helps to explain the paradox outlined above: why a disease of development often most harms those who derive the least benefit from economic booms. This paradox is now playing out on a global scale. The environmental justice movement began in the United States as a response to toxic dumping in poor communities of colour. Such injustice has now gone global, with rich countries outsourcing increasingly toxic industry to those countries that can least cope with its human and environmental consequences (Nixon, 2011). The Bhopal disaster of 1984 provides a glimpse of a changing atmosphere of risk. When the Union Carbide pesticide manufacturing plant in that city exploded in December of that year, it killed thousands of humans and livestock within hours. In the aftermath, cancer rates in the exposure area have tripled, according to a longitudinal study by the Indian Council of Medical Research (Sinhal, 2011). Corporate globalization has diluted the power of the nation-state to regulate environmental pollution, while simultaneously limiting the liability of the worst polluters. New nation-state configurations have also transformed the landscape of responsibility for cancer burdens. Thyroid cancer rates have skyrocketed in the aftermath of the Chernobyl reactor explosion in 1986. Ordinarily thyroid cancer is among the most curable forms of the disease, with recurrence only after twenty-five years in most cases. But it also normally afflicts the elderly, so a twenty-five year remission means that most die of natural causes before the cancer would be likely to return. In Chernobyl, many children are now suffering from these cases, and will surely experience recurrence and metastasis once or more in adulthood. The collapse of the USSR has meant that Ukraine must now bear the consequences of consequences of Soviet negligence, which grossly encumber the country's modest budget (Petryna, 2002).

THE BODY AS ENVIRONMENT

When the Zika virus erupted in headlines in early 2016, it appeared to be a quintessentially tropical disease. Its vector, the *Aedes aegypti* mosquito, is a tropical native with a limited geographic range. Zika had been discovered in Uganda in 1947, and all known subsequent cases had been acquired in tropical settings. If the disease were therefore an environmental hazard linked to the tropics or subtropical settings, exposure would be largely limited to those areas and vulnerable populations within them. But a remarkable op-ed in the *New York Times* in August 2016 put the geography of Zika in a new light. Researchers had established months earlier that the virus was sexually transmissible as well as vector-borne. As Kelly McBride Folkers argued, this forced an important reconsideration of Zika's environment. 'This is not some tropical infection that matters only abroad,' she noted. Instead, 'we should view it more as an S.T.D. that any of us could catch' (Folkers, 2016). That is, because of its sexual transmissibility, Zika's environment was now less the tropics than it was the human body itself. Far from being a disease confined to the tropics, Zika is a disease confined only to the climate of the human body.

There is a bit of sensationalism in Folkers's argument – Zika is unlikely to become the HIV of its era for a number of reasons. But Folkers indicates that while infectious diseases (like cancer) have critical environmental determinants, they also implicate another sense of environment. Their landscape of activity – the environment in which they operate – is the human body. In the course of the twentieth century, the notion of the body as an environment in itself has taken on new and evolving meanings. Just as bodies live and interact in their surroundings, they are also permeable entities that are constructed through their environments. And just as the broader environment is increasingly an anthropogenic space, so too is the body.

The idea of the body as an environment in its own right – as opposed to an entity living in symbiosis with an exterior environment – has a long history.

Although it predates bacteriological theories of contagion and infection, the advent of germ theories paved the way for the 'seed and soil' metaphor that constituted the body as environment in one particular way. If bacteria (and later viruses) were seeds of a sort, they could only take root in an appropriate soil: a susceptible human body. This notion helped to make sense of why some suffered more from disease than others, fitting neatly with degeneration theories of the nineteenth century to explain the stratification of health along class lines (Worboys, 2000). The concept also facilitated ideas about racial disparities of health. Later in the twentieth century, Nazi theorists extended the concept of differential bodily environments to their research on cancer. While they developed extensive research on carcinogenic environmental factors, they also produced extensive theories about genetic and racial determinants of cancer vulnerability as they constantly sought evidence that proved a pathological Jewish inferiority (Proctor, 1999).

Patrick Manson, the founder of the London School of Hygiene and Tropical Medicine, took this idea in a different direction in a series of lectures at Cooper Medical College in San Francisco in 1905. Manson argued that while virtually all flora and fauna are limited in their geographic range by climate and environment, the opposite was true of most pathogens. This is because 'there is practically no variation in the climatic conditions nor in the soil in which they live; for their world, their climate and soil, is the human body with its practically uniform temperature and its practically uniform pabulum'. Manson went on to make what seem like remarkably progressive claims about such human 'uniformity', arguing that 'there is no difference between the juices and tissues of an Esquimaux and those of a Caucasian; or those of a negro; or of those of any given individual of any of these several races' (Manson, 1905). A parasite native to temperate climates could easily live in a human body transplanted to the tropics, and vice versa, as the environment of disease is that of the body, rather than that of its surroundings. While exposure to a given hazard might be limited, vulnerability is universal, a function of the equality of human frailties.

Yet Manson almost immediately walked back his assertions about the universality of human vulnerability. He spends much of the first lecture in a discussion of ankylostomiasis (or hookworm) and its ecology. The disease involves a soil-borne parasite native to warm climates that penetrates the skin and infects the intestines, often causing pernicious anaemia in the patient. It relies on a tropical ecology for infection: the parasite can only live in a warm environment, and usually infects the patient by penetrating the skin of bare feet in contact with the soil. In a discussion of prevention of the disease, Manson cites the example of a plantation owner in Trinidad whose labourers suffered from hookworm infection. The planter had witnessed farmers marching their geese through a pit of tar and then through sand before walking them to market:

the practice created a durable coating that protected their feet from cracking along the way. The planter did the same with his workers, achieving an 'excellent' result: 'coolie itch and coolie anemia almost disappeared from the plantation' (Manson, 1905). The body may be a uniform incubator of disease, but exposure to nature's hazards has been anything but. Vulnerability was the product of a body that was an anthropogenic environment, in which the political economy of plantation labour could alter the body's exposure and resilience.

Just as the racial body constituted different types of environments – whether through heredity or political economy – so too has the body-as-environment been profoundly gendered. While political modernity has often naturalized women's bodies, thereby situating them in close proximity to a specific environment, the consideration of women's bodies as environments has taken on other important meanings in the nineteenth and twentieth centuries. The ecocritic Karen Kilcup has argued that 'the body is women's first environment': the bodies of labouring women, and in particular those of women of colour, have historically constituted a resource to be exploited in a patriarchal society (Kilcup, 2013). The pregnant body also constitutes a specific kind of environment: one that surrounds the foetus, and which is subject to social and political regulation, either through abortion prohibitions or through conventions surrounding diet and behaviours during pregnancy. Links between the contamination of the pregnant body through unhealthy consumption or exposure to toxins and poor health outcomes for children frame the body-as-environment in a way that places important burdens of responsibility on women (Landecker, 2011; Lappé, 2016; Shostak, 2013). The emerging notion of epigenetics and inheritance magnifies this burden, as it implies that corruption of the maternal body-environment will extend to future generations (Landecker and Panofsky, 2013).

The anxieties surrounding pregnant women's bodies as precarious environments underscores the anthropogenic dimensions of this problem. Bodies are manipulable environments subject to human intervention and easily polluted into decay. But twentieth-century medicine has also seen the manipulation of the body's environment as a desired goal. Both allopathic and homeopathic medicine engage in this practice to rid the body of disease, while framing different kinds of bodies as different kinds of environments. If hormones governed women's nature, as Nancy Langston has argued, then modern medicine sought to tame that 'unruly, disordered hormonal environment' through the use of endocrine disrupters (Langston, 2010). The allergic body was another particularly fragile ecology: the development of antihistamines promised to render it resilient to outside forces (Mitman, 2007).

By the turn of the twenty-first century, scientists and patient-advocates alike have begun to imagine the body – like the environment – as a 'site of bio-accumulation', to use the sociologist Martine Lappé's words (Lappé, 2016). Exposures to environmental toxins pollute and transform the body much as lead and arsenic contaminate soil and plastic clogs the oceans, and in just as ineradicable a way. Rachel Carson's *Silent Spring* drew parallels between the accumulation of toxins in the physical environment as well as the body in the early 1960s, establishing a paradigm for the study of the relationships between these forms of contamination. Such accumulation can be accidental, acquired through exposure to contaminants such as carcinogens and endocrine disrupters in polluted water and soil, or it can be intentional, as many in the anti-vaccine movement have argued; for the latter, the battery of immunizations that physicians recommend constitute an overwhelming pollution of children's pristine bodies (Conis, 2014).

The notion of the body as a collector or reservoir of human-made chemicals becomes more complex when considering the body as a repository of living matter as well. While many lament (rightly or wrongly) the accumulation of chemical traces in the body, by the turn of the millennium many microbiome researchers lamented the purification of the body through antibiotic overuse and increasingly sanitized living environments. The human body contains trillions of bacteria on its surface and deep in its core, which perform functions critical to health, bio-absorption and digestion. Yet just as the exploitive practices of industrial society have crushed biodiversity in the natural world, so too have the hygienic practices of modern societies in the global North assaulted

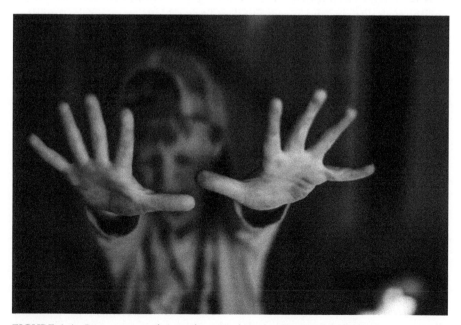

FIGURE 1.4: Recent research into the microbiome suggests that the body is an environment constituted by trillions of beneficial bacteria. Credit: Annie Otzen / Getty Images.

the biodiversity of human microflora, with profound health consequences. In the twentieth century, the use of antibiotics and antibacterial cleansers, suburban houses with purified air systems that are shrink-wrapped with vapour barriers and the processing of food had all long been associated with improving public health. Yet now many argue that these phenomena have been too successful at limiting human microbial exposure, with deleterious effects. Antibiotics have created the phenomenon of *C. diff.*, a highly resistant gut bacterium that causes widespread intestinal misery. They have also correlated closely with an obesity epidemic in the United States. Increasingly sterile domestic spaces may have been responsible for the polio epidemics of the mid-twentieth century and for rising rates of allergy and asthma in the present. Researchers have proposed probiotics, fermented foods, playing and working outside, faecal transplants and adding a dog to the family as possible mechanisms for restoring a healthy ecology of the body (Pollan, 2013; Klass, 2017).

CONCLUSIONS

Many twentieth-century ideas about the intersection of environment and health are now undergoing profound revision. Researchers have now labelled a number of infectious diseases as carcinogenic. The American chemical industry attacked Rachel Carson viciously for drawing connections between exposure to environmental toxins and cancer in *Silent Spring*. Now, many on the American Right accuse her of causing the global malaria pandemic, as her work contributed to bans on the use of DDT to kill mosquitoes. The antiseptic environment that was an ideal of the late twentieth century has now proven treacherous to the human microbiome: the quest for a clean environment has now transformed into a desire for a dirty body.

Yet through this enormous flux, the question of exposure and vulnerability remains constant. Hazards persist in every environment, yet not everyone is equally exposed or equally vulnerable. Vulnerability and resilience often track along socioeconomic status, but not always, as diseases have specific forms of agency: Lyme disease and certain cancers give the lie to the notion that illness is necessarily a function of inequality. Yet in most cases, an environmental justice of sickness and health places the burden most profoundly on those who share the fewest benefits of global economic growth.

Ecological interpretations of disease as a function of the relationship between people and their surroundings are not new. In the early and mid-twentieth century, scientists such as Hans Zinsser, Macfarlane Burnet and Frank Fenner sought to avoid what they saw as the facile reductionism of germ theories of disease to advance more complex ideas about the interactions of microbes with their hosts and their environments (Anderson, 2004). In the 2000s, the OneHealth movement advocated for an integrative ecosystem approach to health and disease that emphasizes the interconnection of human, animal and environmental health. The latter movement self-consciously presented itself as the heir to a Hippocratic tradition that seeks the preservation of health through a broader environmental consciousness.

What I am advocating here is something slightly different. I argue that we must see 'environment' not merely as the situatedness of people in the world, but as a product of human social and natural relations, with each other and their surroundings. Environmental crisis, by this reading, is not merely something like unsustainable livestock rearing practices (as a OneHealth practitioner might argue), but also the defunding of public education and neighbourhood decline (DiChiro, 1995). Environmental sustainability is not merely mindful consumption and careful stewardship of resources, but also the cultivation of sociability (Keller, 2015). Changes in behaviour alter sociability in ways that transform human as well as human-nonhuman interaction, and therefore change local ecologies, creating new susceptibilities as well as forms of resilience. As the ecocritic Robert Nixon has argued, 'We may all be in the Anthropocene but we're not all in it in the same way' (Nixon, 2014). This chapter argues that such an insight applies as well to the relationships among sickness, health and the environment. While hazards are everywhere, exposures to them, as well as consequent vulnerabilities, are unequal and often unpredictable.

CHAPTER TWO

Food

NANCY N. CHEN

In the second decade of the twenty-first century, upscale North American and European supermarkets might include shelves stocked with bone broth, fermented foods or probiotic drinks. These items join a growing list of super foods and other functional foods that are promoted to consumers pursuing the latest food fad or dietary advice by health websites, weight loss guides, fitness trainers or food experts. Food markets across Asia filled with growing middle-class consumers in China and India also carry the latest health food items that cater to local preferences such as nutraceutical food products or vitamin enhanced baby water. Such products reflect the transformation of industrialized food systems to incorporate medicinal food practices into everyday forms of consumption. Contemporary food marketers increasingly look to traditional medicines and global health foods to seek out innovative products that may invigorate a multinational food or beverage conglomerate's sales across regional markets. Substances such as turmeric may be simultaneously considered to be a spice, dietary supplement, medicinal food or beverage source such that a retail outlet might carry turmeric in these multiple forms across different sections of the same store. These material entities and their diverse mercantile categorization reflect long-standing cultural frameworks of food and medicine as well as contemporary legal contexts and marketing practices. How might these formations reflect the role of food in framing notions of health, nutrition or disease?

In this chapter, I examine shifting categories of food, dietary therapy and medicine during the twentieth century, which extends well into the present. Though food and medicine have been intertwined for many centuries, throughout the twentieth century the long-standing emphasis on preventative medicine through food and diet as beneficial gave way to concerns about food as worrisome even dangerous risks to health. How did notions of food as medicine and dietary therapy become separate spheres of healing from biomedical practice? Eating and medicating became distinct practices and categories despite long multicultural traditions of consuming medicinal foods, especially herbs and spices as integral to healing. This chapter will examine the tensions inherent in maintaining these separate categories, specifically through their governance, and how food remains integral to the study of health and biomedicine.

The first part of this chapter will address the transformation from food *as* medicine to food *and* medicine as distinct spheres. During the mid-twentieth century, the rise of the pharmaceutical industry emphasized the separation of food and medicine with scientific discoveries of vitamins, vaccines and other products became industrialized into pharmaceutical products. These forms of biomedicine shaped modern notions of embodiment and nutrition with distinct bodily ideals and dietary practices. Along with the shift from primary care in small clinical practices to tertiary care in hospitals with the professionalization of medical practitioners, dietary changes from transformations in agriculture and the development of global food chains deepened the chasm between food and biomedicine. The politics of ingestion and digestion frame the second part of this discussion. In the late twentieth century, interest in holistic and alternative medicine revived theories of classical medicine and dietary therapy as consumers avidly pursued these therapeutic modalities even paying out of pocket when insurance did not cover these forms. Following popular interest in complementary medicine, the food industry developed new assemblages of medicinal food and dietary therapy in the form of nutraceuticals. Notions of balance, in particular, will be explored in this latter half of the chapter as dietary regimens focus on functional foods, gut-brain connectivity and ethical contexts of eating. Food remains foundational for both disease and wellness. The pendulum for defining well-being has renewed notions of food *as* medicine through rethinking notions of digestion, dietary standards and food safety.

BIOMEDICAL AND NUTRITIONAL WORLDS
OF THE TWENTIETH CENTURY

Multiple streams of medicinal beliefs and healthy foods circulated during the early twentieth century as an extension of health reform movements prominent during the latter half of the nineteenth century. In the transition from religious doctrines about eating as holiness to secular views of bodies and notions of hygiene, the focus on digestion to promote better health became part of medical practice. Dietary regimens were deemed crucial to maintaining bodily balance and homeostatic equilibrium between consumption and elimination. Processing food took place not only within the digestive tract but also outside the human body prior to ingestion with the production of new forms of food such as processed grains as breakfast cereals. Timing was just as important as what food was to be eaten. Specific formulations on the proper consumption of foods at particular times became part of dietary advice that were being practised at health spas and clinics in Europe as well as the notable Battle Creek Sanitarium in the United States (Bauch, 2017). Such practices continued to maintain the intimate connection between food and medicine similar to classical formulations of medicine with food being the frontline of treating disease. What followed for the majority of the twentieth century, however, was the eventual separation of food and medicine into distinct spheres with the industrialization of both agriculture and biomedicine.

The gradual emergence of the United States Food and Drug Administration (FDA) as a 'scientific, regulatory, and public health agency' offers insight onto the circuitous path of governance over food and medicine during this period. Initially located in the Department of Agriculture with a sole chemist as its employee in the nineteenth century during the Civil War, the agency moved to the Division and then Bureau of Chemistry at the onset of the twentieth century. It was the penultimate federal Food and Drugs Act of 1906 that gave this entity a regulatory role. This history is narrated in the following passage from the agency's website:

> Beginning as the Division of Chemistry and then (after July 1901) the Bureau of Chemistry, the modern era of the FDA dates to 1906 with the passage of the Federal Food and Drugs Act; this added regulatory functions to the agency's scientific mission. The Bureau of Chemistry's name changed to the Food, Drug, and Insecticide Administration in July 1927, when the non-regulatory research functions of the bureau were transferred elsewhere in the department. In July 1930 the name was shortened to the present version. FDA remained under the Department of Agriculture until June 1940, when the agency was moved to the new Federal Security Agency. In April 1953 the agency again was transferred, to the Department of Health, Education, and Welfare (HEW). Fifteen years later FDA became part of the Public Health Service within HEW, and in May 1980 the education function was removed from HEW to create the Department of Health and Human Services, FDA's current home. To understand the development of this agency is to understand the laws it regulates, how the FDA has administered these laws, how the courts have interpreted the legislation, and how major events have driven all three.
>
> —Swann on FDA Origins referring to Kurian, 1998

Since its inception, the mission of the FDA was revised in subsequent decades with amendments to coordinate with federal law and interagency oversight.

The regulatory powers of the agency were further expanded with the congressional Federal Food, Drug, and Cosmetic Act of 1938, which authorized now standard factory inspections, premarket safety approval, false claim prohibition, proper labelling and jurisdiction over cosmetics and medical devices in addition to foods and medicines. Initially featuring sample food

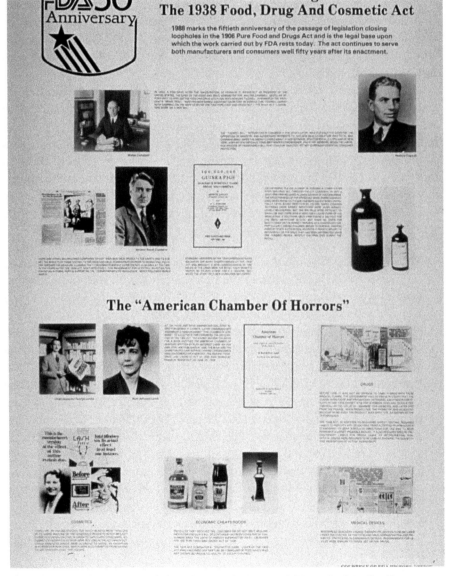

FIGURE 2.1: The securing of the 1938 Food, Drug and Cosmetic Act. Credit: National Library of Medicine.

products to illustrate the need for standards, the 1933 exhibit took on the title 'American Chamber of Horrors' after a news article on the topic. Many of the items included popular foods at the time and well-known labels to illustrate to Congress the need for consumers to identify easily quality and expense with accurate labelling, packaging and descriptions. The exhibit was displayed not only at the White House but also later at the Chicago World's Fair in the same year. The fiftieth anniversary of the Act was commemorated with an official poster that includes some of the items from the exhibit.

As Carpenter notes in his analysis on history of the FDA, the regulatory structure and influence of the agency is framed by the systematic creation and engagement of particular 'audiences' which might consist of scientific and professional organizations, academic institutions, or private firms (Carpenter, 2014: 33). By adopting definitions and concepts from the FDA, the governing agency gathers recognition and authority to regulate. Moreover, such concerned audience members become extensions of the regulatory process as these parties engage with its policies. The shift from being under the umbrella of the Department of Agriculture to the Department of Health, moreover, reflected the growing role of this agency in monitoring and governing of the rising pharmaceutical industry.

The decades leading up to the Second World War were filled with multiple scientific discoveries and technologies that remain influential for present-day biomedicine. In addition to the identification of vitamins, vaccines and insulin, new medical devices such as the electrocardiogram or the isolation of drugs such as penicillin came to be produced for commercial purposes. The rise of the pharmaceutical industry consolidated two streams of practice: late nineteenth-century apothecaries that became wholesale suppliers for drug manufacturing in addition to chemists isolating specific compounds initially from plant- and animal-based products to created concentrated forms. As chemical companies embarked on creating synthetic forms for medicinal use, local pharmacists continued to create compounds for medicine (Dammreich and Bowden, 2005). The pharmaceutical industry rose to greater prominence in industrialized countries during wartime, which continued in the post-Second World War era. The need for penicillin, antimalarial drugs and antibiotics, in particular, contributed to the expansion for pharmaceutical pipelines of research, development and marketing across the US, Europe and Japan. The influence of biomedicine extended well beyond industrialized nations to colonialized regions of Africa and Asia as well as other nation-states during the early twentieth century.

As overlapping realms of experimental lab science, drug development, clinical research and pharmacy storefronts emerged in the post-war context, accompanying professional associations and disciplines began to claim expertise and stake ownership over areas of medical knowledge. Dumit's documentation of prescription drugs and their ubiquity in everyday life in the US suggests that pharmaceutical interventions into scientific research, health care provision and even mass marketing have not only been normalized but have also spawned new assemblages of expectation, demand and consumption on the part of consumer patients (Dumit, 2012). These formations of knowledge and the material forms facilitated processes of worldmaking or worlding that shape notions of disease and cure in biomedicine as well as its alternatives (Zhan, 2009). The twentieth century can thus be considered as the everlasting pharmaceutical century with the phenomenal rise of the drug industry and randomized drug trials that are global in reach and infrastructure (Dumit, 2012; Lakoff, 2006; Petryna, 2005). The biomedicalization of everyday life through drugs prescribed to counter deadly illnesses, foods measured in units to promote weight loss, and regulatory structures aimed at preventing fraud shaped the worlds of food and medicine throughout the long twentieth century. Pharmacovigilance, the careful monitoring and assessment of drugs for adverse effects after release to consumers, remains a key concern for everyday life not only with prescribed and over-the-counter drugs, but also for unauthorized uses of such drugs and other illicit substances which have become a grave concern worldwide (Langlitz, 2009). Such concerns shape not only pharmaceutical drugs but also forms of dietary and nutritional supplementation.

While the pharmaceutical industry reframed categories of food and medicine into distinct realms, the discovery of thirteen vitamins with advancements in biochemistry research during the first half of the twentieth century introduced the concept of micronutrients in dietary metabolism and health. Historical observations of nutrition deficiency based diseases such as scurvy, beriberi, rickets, goitre and pellagra among sailors and vulnerable captive or prison populations subjected to food deprivation emphasized the significant impact of dietary deficiency. The isolation and identification of vitamins in laboratory science was translated into domestic spheres through lessons on child rearing and early nutrition. The connection of vitamins with certain foods formed the basis of dietary lessons given to children and parents during wartime and throughout the Cold War era.

In addition to women and children as key audiences for these new techniques of cooking and nutritional management, males in the industrial workforce and military were also deemed critical targets of nutritional consumption, as seen in the poster by the U.S. Public Health Service which highlights foods to 'Keep men strong and on the job'.

Vitamins were believed to restore vital energy to foods lost in cooking or other forms of processing leading to the insertion of vitamins into food products. The enrichment of foods with micronutrients was used not only to replace nutrients lost in processing but also to increase trace amounts to enhance nutritional quality. In the post-war context, the key audience

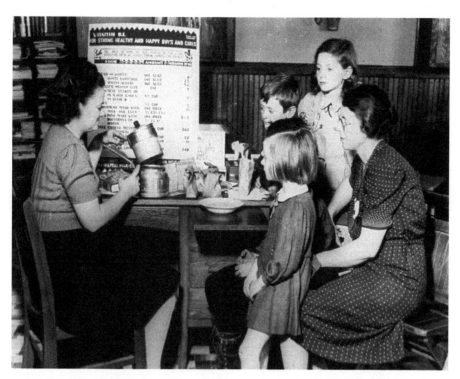

FIGURE 2.2: Image from the Children's Bureau of a mother with four children observing demonstration of cooking utensil for steaming food next to large poster about vitamin B. Credit: National Library of Medicine/ United States Children's Bureau.

shifted from families and working men to children as new consumers. Vitamin supplementation was introduced with advertising as a necessary step towards securing an adequate diet and better health. The scientific discovery of vitamins quickly transformed into middle-class standards of child rearing by the mid-twentieth century. Annual medical exams of children included recommendations for vitamin consumption as notions of insufficiency continued to shape notions of bodies in this period.

The story of public health during this period tends to narrate success in overcoming infectious diseases and increased mortality as a result of new discoveries in vaccines and the onward progress of science and modernization. However, the rise in lifespans and decreased infant mortality were actually reflections of better nutrition and promotion of primary health care and disease prevention. The discovery of folate, a water-soluble vitamin, and its synthetic form of folic acid as possibly reducing cases of neural tube disorders in newborns eventually led to the widespread fortification of flour and cereal grains. Moreover, folic acid in prenatal vitamins was prescribed to women both prior to conception and during pregnancy (Crider et al., 2011; Junod, 2001). While

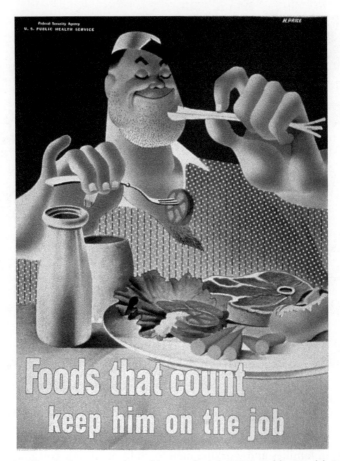

FIGURE 2.3: "Foods that count: keep him on the job," U.S. Public Health Service Poster, 1942. Credit: National Library of Medicine/U.S. Public Health Service.

folate is abundant in leafy green vegetables, both fortification (the addition of micronutrients into food) and biofortification (the modification of food crops for higher yield) came to be technological fixes for addressing public health needs, especially for women and children in developing nations (Kimura, 2013). Beyond public health, vitamin and mineral supplements, especially multivitamin tablets, became part of middle-class practices of self-care and daily life. Rather than consuming a range of foods to ensure adequate nutritional intake, the consumption of vitamins became encouraged as part of regular health maintenance. Vitamins fitted easily into everyday life as part of the continuum of taking pills. Whether in wellness or in illness, there was a pill either as a supplement or as a cure. Dietary supplements in the latter part of the twentieth century quickly grew to a multibillion-dollar industry, especially since these were regulated not as drugs but as food.

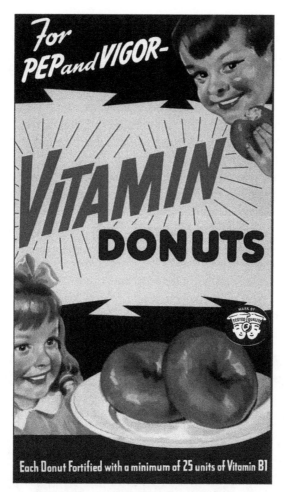

FIGURE 2.4: Vitamin B Donuts. Credit: Wikimedia Commons/U.S. Food and Drug Administration.

Figure 2.4 shows a 1941 product from the Donut Corporation of America that was proposed to the wartime Nutrition Division. The inclusion of enriched flour as the main ingredient supplying vitamin B was not sufficient for the government to approve the advertising campaign for the product. While the vitamin B donut was not approved to be mass produced, the promotion of fortified foods was taken up again at the end of the twentieth century as nutraceuticals.

In other areas of scientific research, foods came to be considered as forms of energy to fuel essential bodily functions and maintenance. The notion of calorie initially emerged in the nineteenth century as part of French popular physics that became translated into German physiology and eventually American nutrition. Over several decades, the physical notion of how much energy was needed to heat a kilogram of water by one degree Celsius gave way to nutritional notions of calories as forms of measurement to be used in dietetics (Hargrove, 2006). The terms for calorie in chemistry is usually designated by the lower case letter 'c' while the nutritional term kilojoule is used interchangeable with kilocalorie or Calorie, spelled with the upper case 'C' to distinguish the nutritional context. In everyday usage, however, most popular mediums of information tend to use the terms interchangeably. By the start of the twentieth century, the quantification of calories facilitated the role of scientific measurement in the realm of nutrition (Mudry, 2009). In this new realm of food management, dietitians became experts in interpreting how caloric intake could shape the trajectory of a disease or the impact of dietary knowledge on health outcome.

Initially framed by dietitians at mid-century, focus on caloric intake came to be part of everyday concerns for proper dietary consumption. Together with changes in labelling laws, ordinary consumers became avid readers of nutrition labels for content and caloric intake. Calories came to be considered something to be managed as concerns for obesity and other chronic health conditions shifted towards weight management and loss as part of disease prevention, especially for the growing middle classes (Gilman, 2008).

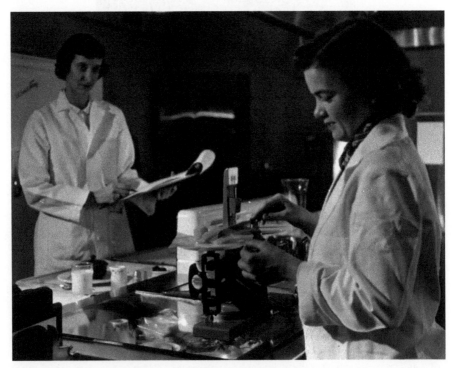

FIGURE 2.5: Two female dieticians weigh and measure foods before they are served to patients of restrictive diets. Credit: National Library of Medicine.

Throughout the twentieth century, but especially in the latter half, the emergence of the food industry with political lobbyists to procure influence in US government policy began to shift beliefs from eating more food during food shortages and wartime rationing to the notion of 'eating less' as Nestle documents in her study of the American food industry (2002). With growing rates of chronic disorders such as cardiovascular disease, diabetes and obesity, certain foods were believed to contribute to long-term morbidity of such diseases. Not unlike early twentieth-century views about meat and alcohol as unhealthy and the promotion of abstinence from such substances, the view that certain food ingredients such as fats, sugar and (more recently) gluten were unhealthy led to secular taboos or negative connotations of these ingredients.

The introduction of foods as dangerous or health risks facilitated the growth of dietary fads that took two directions. One trend illustrates Dupuis' notion of 'ingestive subjectivity' (2015: 7), whereby individuals choose to consume carefully in order to prevent threats or dangerous foods from entering their body. Harm, and, by extension, chronic disease, could be preventable by consuming health foods, such as granola or brown rice. The emergence of health foods during the 1960s and 1970s in the West was contiguous with counter-culture movements, cooperative enterprises and environmental consciousness during that period. A different trajectory of the concerns for dangerous foods leading to chronic disease was the expansion of the diet industry, which emphasized slim body image and body weight as the way to health. Special dieting programmes and affiliated products such as books, tapes, special diet foods, weight loss clinics, fitness programmes and dieting experts abounded with the ever growing concerns of the middle class and elites concerned with expanding waistlines. Dimorphic, gendered notions of idealized bodies for males and females betweeen the 1970s and 1990s underscored overall emphasis on appearance that promoted eating less. It is not surprising that diagnoses of eating disorders such as anorexia nervosa and bulimia also grew significantly during this time. Counting calories and consuming special diet foods initially became part of daily life for groups concerned with weight management such as athletes, entertainers, elites and women. With the continued rise of processed foods, ubiquity of cheap fast foods, expansion of the global food chain and food deserts, chronic conditions related to excess weight such as obesity, diabetes, cardiovascular disease and circulatory problems have spread beyond the middle classes. In many parts of the world, it is the working poor and children who currently face obesogenic conditions whether by residing in food deserts with limited access to fresh and nutritious foods or not being able to afford healthy foods and lifestyles (Guthman, 2011). New populations of risk have been targeted not only by public health programmes but also by the expanding food industry, which seeks emerging markets and cultivates new consumers with their brands. Food scholars and activists have

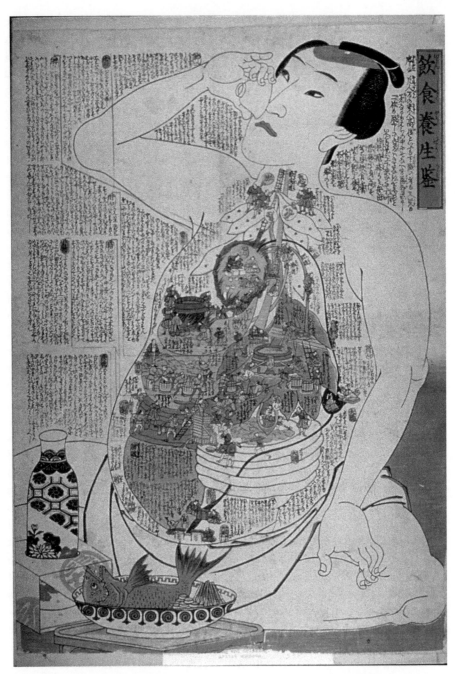

FIGURE 2.6: Inshoku yōjō kagami, circa 1890. Japanese print illustrating the
functions of the digestive system and other internal organs of a man whose body is
shown with the organs displayed. Within each organ, small people help to perform the
various bodily functions. The man sits before a bowl of food and sips tea. Credit:
National Library of Medicine.

drawn attention to the social justice dimensions of food access and consumption to contextualize better the epidemiological patterns and statistics for chronic disease. While the introduction of micronutrients and biofortification into processed foods has been promoted by international development projects as solutions for feeding populations at risk, these measures highlight the role of technoscientific expertise while de-emphasizing the role of women as knowledgeable agents in food security and providing nutritious meals (Kimura, 2013). Moreover, the study of how food comes to be associated with love, blame or shame is just as relevant in both emerging economies and prosperous regions (Solomon, 2016).

The expansion of the global food chain in the twentieth century is also a critical factor in the transformation from foods as medicinal into foods as commodities. Over the past two decades, food scholars and activists have turned the lens back onto food systems which globalized dramatically with extensive market chains that transported fresh produce and tropical fruits from Africa and Latin America to the markets of Europe and middle-class retail grocery stores of North America and Asia (Friedberg, 2014). The global desire for sushi has created new commodity chains for tuna and other raw fish not only for consumers in Japan but worldwide (Bestor, 2004). The extensive distance and time required to facilitate a global summer filled with unseasonal foods require considerable investments in the form of harvest labour, packaging, refrigeration, shipping, retail marketing and advertising. Such cash crops also transform local landscapes by taking land formerly used for diverse subsistence food crops for monocropping or worse, in doing so, rendering such lands unusable due to toxic build-up after using fertilizers, pesticides and other chemicals (Muenster, 2015). The longer distances that foods travel deepen the carbon footprint of the food industry. Despite transformations in refrigeration and transportation technology that enable foods to move very swiftly and retain a semblance of freshness, the nutritional value of foods decreases with every additional step of processing and travel. While the organic food movement has embraced foods sourced locally and grown without pesticides, significant concerns remain about food justice in terms of who gets access to such foods. Agricultural labourers grow, harvest and bring such crops to the table often at great personal risk and amidst health concerns (Holmes, 2014; Horton, 2016).

The recognition of the impact of food on both well-being and disease profoundly shaped the medicinal and nutritional worlds of the twentieth century. In what follows, I address how the epidemiological transition from acute infectious diseases to chronic conditions influenced the search for new frameworks of medical foodways that could be effective for diseases such as cardiovascular disease, hypertension or diabetes.

BACK TO THE FUTURE? FUNCTIONAL FOODS

During the 1990s, new forms of medicinal foodways or combinations of food and medicine emerged. Researchers found that certain elements of the foods consumed for health reasons could be extracted from various plants and put into pills or powders and combined with food items. These entities were called nutraceuticals (from nutrition and pharmaceutical) or also referred to as functional foods: food and drinks with physiological effects that may help reduce chronic disease. Over the past two decades, the nutraceutical industry has developed a wide range of products to meet growing interest from consumers. Nutraceuticals reframe key questions about medicine as food. Are these superfoods enhanced with fortified compounds or just dietary supplements in food form rather than pills? Though conventional food and medicine are considered to be separate categories, new technologies are enabling novel forms of eating and drinking one's way to health.

Nutraceuticals range from foods in recognizable forms such as garlic or grapes to more bioengineered foods that have isolated compounds or supplements. Food science scholars further elaborate, 'Nutraceuticals are naturally-derived, bioactive (usually phytochemical) compounds that have health promoting, disease preventing or medicinal properties' (Lachance and Saba, 2002). The category of enriched foods or medicines consumed in the form of food is a booming industry. Omega three-enriched eggs, vitamin-enriched drinks or calcium supplements in the form of chocolate are all readily available in markets. Together with the ubiquity of food supplements and the pharmaceutical industry established at mid-century, nutraceuticals permeate daily life.

Functional foods are designed to have specific health-promoting functions. For instance, garlic compounds are believed to be useful to lower hypertension, prevent cardiovascular heart disease and even prevent or treat cancer. The association of lycopene, a carotenoid found in tomatoes, with the reduction of cancer cells has boosted the consumption of tomato-based foods. While the FDA has ruled that food manufacturers may not overtly promote a product as cancer-reducing, research on this topic has continued to be pursued by the food industry. The term 'functional foods' may also refer to unmodified foods. However, genetically engineered and vitamin-fortified foods have also been considered to be functional foods as well.

For many consumers, nutraceuticals might be considered an extension of vitamins. Rather than consuming a vitamin separately or in with one's food, nutraceutical products are packaged as convenient additives and even delicious ways to enhance one's health. However, nutraceuticals differ from vitamins in that some products include items that may not occur as natural substances. Considerable efforts have been made to isolate compounds such as flavonoids (water-soluble plant pigments) that can be found in chocolate, wine, tea, strawberries or raisins. Flavonoid-rich foods have been associated with beneficial cardiovascular effects. But the direct connection between flavonoid-enhanced foods and improved cardiovascular health has not been proven. The category of nutraceuticals draws on notions of natural foods; however, the isolation of a compound to infuse a food through industrial processing is quite different from foods found in nature. Depending upon the food or drink product, the role of the nutraceutical tends to be featured as a valuable additive which heightens the value and therefore cost of the original food item, not unlike the 1941 vitamin B donut advertisement addressed in the previous section.

As the nutraceutical industry expands worldwide, questions of audience and access arise. Paying close attention to who produces, buys and consumes nutraceuticals continues to be critical elements for industrial firms as well as their governance by state agencies. With the development of such products as capital-intensive enterprises, the issue of how nutraceuticals reaches consumers entails a regulatory dance between producers and governing agencies. Will nutraceuticals follow the likely trajectory of organic foods, which tend to be directed at the high end of markets, or will these products be made available to consumers of different economic backgrounds? As more nutraceutical products become available in local groceries, knowledge about nutrition on the part of consumers will also shape the integration of these products into everyday life. The nutraceutical industry faces ongoing work to develop nutritional standards. Concerns for quality management, standardization and substantiation of claims reflect similar concerns with dietary supplements. As a category, nutraceuticals have been transformed by various stakeholders: the industrial food system, pharmaceutical industry, government regulators, international classification systems and, not least, consumers. Shaping the tastes of consumers for nutraceuticals often entails masking the medicine-like herbal taste associated with many health drinks or blending specific nutrients with foods that are already appealing, such as chocolate. The taste of nutraceuticals, like medicine, continues to be dominated by sweetness and neoliberal framings of food and medicine as commodities. Rather than consider functional foods as the return of medicinal foodways in the late twentieth century, their formation as products to be procured, processed and sold in markets reflects how foods, diets and medicines have come to be defined by capitalism and neoliberal policies. In many ways, the incorporation of nutraceuticals into daily consumption, whether as a supplement, beverage, snack or new menu item, reflects how notions of nutrition have evolved throughout the twentieth century. Particularly at the end of the century, the tremendous rise in different forms of dietary practices offer insight onto nutritional regimes as self technologies to shape bodies, minds and communities. Functional foods complete the trajectory that vitamins offered at mid-century by shaping food categories that have particular nutritional values or capacities, and yet are somehow deficient without additional supplementation.

Moreover, nutraceuticals enable consumers to choose in what forms and at what times such additions are made. In what follows, I address how such vastly changing ecologies and knowledge concerning diet and nutrition shift the focus from the governance of food and drug categories as separate spheres to their integration in reframing overall well-being.

RECONNECTING BODIES, ENVIRONMENTS, HEALTH AND CULTURE THROUGH FOOD

In the new millennium, the role of diet and food as central to the consideration of health has evolved in several ways. The dangers of eating not only encompass concerns for obesity but also allergies and food sensitivities that grown significantly during the twenty-first century. Bodies are perceived as increasingly out of balance due to exposure to dramatic changes to the nexus of air, water and soil. Foods directly convey these multiple forms of exposure through consumption at any point in a food chain, whether by insects, animals or humans (Landeker, 2011). New worlds of risk emerge in this context, ranging from more exceptional forms such as radiation exposure, toxic waste and chemical overload to normalized everyday experiences of urban pollution, lead exposure, carcinogenic agents and viral outbreaks. These configurations of exposure reveal complicated stories of risk that integrate human bodies with the health of other species as well as damaged environments. In moving away from the modern era as a period that emphasized formal scientific and technological progress, the move towards consideration of deeper connections between nature, society and politics has renewed focus on ecological systems of food and medicine. The reconnection of these two realms offers more complex possibilities than merely the production of functional foods addressed in the previous section. In the following, I address key arenas where rethinking the connections between guts and brains as well as genes and the environment facilitate new directions in the understanding of food, dietary practices and health.

Though knowledge of microorganisms within human bodies emerged during the late nineteenth century, recent exploration of the human microbiome since 2007 has transformed contemporary views of the body and physiological functions. Multiple forms of diverse microorganisms, including trillions of bacterial communities, reside within human tissue and contribute towards key functions such as digestion, immunity and brain activity. Taking into account how metabolic processes are not only incredibly diverse but also dynamic with dietary, environmental and genomic variation brings forth quite different understandings of human bodies and ongoing transformations. The role of the human gut and its microbiota is perhaps one of the key stories of the present to highlight the influence of diet and metabolism for health in critical new ways.

Fermentation is an age-old technology of using microorganisms such as yeast, bacteria or other microbes to break down substances and transform them into foods such as kimchi, sauerkraut, miso, pickles, yoghurt or sourdough bread, as well as alcoholic beverages such as beer, cider or wine, or other beverages such as kefir or kombucha. The renewal of artisanal food practices such as fermented products has become featured in urban farmers' markets as well as restaurants featuring local foods or farm-to-fork dining. Fermented foods and beverages can be seen not only as traditional functional foods but also as the extension of the microbial environment into the gastrointestinal. In her study on contested framings of raw milk as biohazard or as artisanal food craft, Paxson engages the notion of microbiopolitics to offer expanded notions of nutrition that facilitate heterogeneity in tastes and food preferences rather than modern notions of food safety that determine how one form of microorganism fits all (2014).

The growing research on epigenetics – the influence of environment on how genes get expressed, or not, to influence life functions – is another major pivot point in nutritional science and dietary knowledge. The assemblage of epigenetic knowledge has significant implications for how food and diet influence the outcomes of disease, ageing, obesity or even sleep at cellular levels. Beyond the consideration of digestion and dietary patterns within a single body, researchers are also documenting the effects of epigenetics on longitudinal development and transgenerational inheritance. The concept of plasticity, the ability to change or adapt to new environments, in this new realm reflects how nutrients can have a great impact at microcellular levels.

A growing world population (currently 7 billion) projected to reach 8.5 billion by 2030 offers stark reminders that food security and the equitable distribution of food will continue to be key challenges in this century. Access to food for refugees and military troops often entails foods that are stripped of social context such as bars filled with basic nutrients or ready-meals. Such foods have been extensively processed for long-term shelf life, which tends to be coded as not desirable. Nonetheless, such transportable forms of sustenance illuminate how survival continues to shape when food is a fuel rather than the means for defining belonging and kinship.

Dietary fads in recent years have continued to follow the latest scientific research to address cancer, diabetes or ageing. With ongoing concerns for damaged environments, it is not surprising to find advertisements for new dietary products, vitamins, food supplements and even enriched water with claims that promote safety and well-being. In light of ongoing food scandals and concerns for contaminated foods, even fake foods in some markets, securing the integrity of foods and medicines require both governance for food and drug production and careful scrutiny at the level of consumption.

While the majority of this chapter has focused on the materiality of foods and medicine as well as their governance, in closing it is crucial to return to the moral and symbolic frameworks of food, diet and nutrition. As economic and social anthropologist Sidney Mintz's work on food and culture illustrates, food is indexical of power, class, gender, race and ethnicity (Mintz, 1982). Just as eating and feeding are dense sites of sociality and identity, dietary regimes are also powerful forms of self-making technology and forms of care. Tracking the ways in which the knowledge of how foods may be used as medicines or dietary therapy is also reflective of status, access and belonging. The practice of medicine cannot simply be reduced to physiological measurements such as blood pressure, body temperature or bodily chemistry. As the other chapters in this volume illustrate, medicine is far more nuanced and reflects ongoing socioeconomic transformations as well as political life and cultural practices. The role of food and nutrition is a critical part of both health and disease. Well-being is not merely the consumption of foods and medicines but also the engagement of dietary practices and nutritional knowledge as foundations for overall health.

CHAPTER THREE

Disease

JEREMY A. GREENE

KNOW YOUR SYNDROME: EXPANDING VALENCES OF DISEASE, 1920–2000

In 1919, the Danish physician Knud Faber first published a slim book on *Nosography in Modern Internal Medicine* that made him, at least for a little while, a minor celebrity in the medical world. In it, he argued that the classification of the world of human ailments into a list of specific diseases was one of the central organizing concepts of modern medicine – and perhaps the single most important aspect of medical modernity. 'To the clinician it is essential,' he concluded, as 'he cannot live, speak, or act without the concept of morbid categories' (Faber, 1923, vii). Faber took his readers on a historical tour of the concept of disease as specific entity, from the seventeenth-century nosological listings of Thomas Sydenham through the pathological anatomy of the early nineteenth century Paris Clinic, the development of the physiological and pathological sciences in Germany and France, and the formulation of the germ theory of disease. The work culminated with the broader application of Koch's postulates in the early twentieth century, linking the laboratory and the clinic through causal chains of *in vitro* and *in vivo* proofs of disease and prompting the development of powerful new technologies for the specific diagnosis and treatment of individual diseases.

Faber's book circulated widely: the first run of a 1922 English edition sold out swiftly and was reprinted in 1923, followed by a second edition in 1930. It was especially popular among leaders within the institutions of academic medicine whose achievements it celebrated. Rufus Cole, head of the Rockefeller Institute, claimed that 'one cannot read in these pages the history of the

development of internal medicine without acquiring an increased respect for
this branch of human knowledge, and without being convinced that it will
ultimately rate as a science even if, as some mention, in its present state it does
not deserve a place in that category' (Faber, 1923, ix). Faber's story of the
history of disease was easily digestible for biomedical modernists like Cole: it
was intellectual, teleological, progressive and heroic, and aestheticized medicine
as a pure science at last separable from the cruder art that had encased it for
centuries, like a sculpture of Athena being revealed from a block of raw marble.
Together, Faber, Cole and thousands of other physicians saw a future of
increasingly precise medicine, in which every ailment might have a specific and
knowable cause, course and cure.

The same narrative of medicine as a science whose increasing power to
define and therefore control disease continues to motivate many physicians and
philanthropists in the early twenty-first century. As I sit down to write this
chapter in the fall of 2016, a front-page *Washington Post* article has just detailed
a $3 billion pledge by Facebook billionaires Priscilla Chan and Mark Zuckerberg
to 'cure, prevent, or manage all disease' by the year 2100.[1] Like Faber and
Cole's enthusiasm in the early twentieth century, their optimism is based on the
value of precision, as the National Institutes of Health and most academic
medical centres in North America promise a series of 'remarkable breakthroughs
that represent precision medicine's potential to eliminate human diseases'.[2]
One is tempted simply to connect the dots between Faber and Cole in 1923 and
Chan and Zuckerberg in 2016, and call it progress. But in the century or so in
between, the history of disease has been anything but a straight line.

It is true, as Faber argues, that the sharpening delineation of specific disease
categories had become central to the consolidation of new biomedical forms of
knowledge and practice by the 1920s. Yet the burden of health and disease, the
delineation of normality and pathology, and the methods by which we tell them
apart have continued to transform over the twentieth and twenty-first centuries
in ways that these early twentieth century modernists could not foresee.
Looking at the swelling page count of the World Health Organization's
International Classification of Diseases (now on its eleventh version), or the
rising ranks of children in the US who carry diagnoses of chronic disease before
their tenth birthday, one has to wonder: does twenty-first-century medicine
have any chance to eliminate diseases when it has been so much more successful
at producing new ones? To tell the history of disease in the twentieth and
twenty-first centuries, then, requires a very different mode of storytelling.

THE SHIFTING BURDEN OF DISEASE

If a world free of disease is too much to ask for, then the smaller prospect of a
world without infectious disease, or without a handful of the worst infectious

diseases might seem a more reasonable goal. The promise of disease eradication has motivated several generations of physicians and public health officials over the course of the twentieth and twenty-first centuries. Charles-Edward Amory Winslow, one of the founding members of the Society of American Bacteriologists and the Yale School of Public Health, issued a sort of biomedical promissory note in 1943 when he cheered on 'the consecutive story of an intellectual progress which has made possible one of the greatest practical triumphs in the history of the human race: the conquest of epidemic disease' (Winslow, 1943, xii).

Winslow's *Conquest of Epidemic Disease* was published the same year that penicillin became widely available and concluded with the optimistic statement that 'the practical application of the principles developed by a series of clear thinkers and brilliant investigators – from Fracastorius to Chapin – has forever banished from the earth the major pestilences and plagues of the past' (Winslow, 1944, 380). And if it has recently been revealed that that U.S. Surgeon General William Stewart never did say, in 1967, that 'It's time to close the books on infectious diseases, declare the war against pestilence won, and shift national resources to such chronic problems as cancer and heart disease,' this misattribution has been persistent in part because it captured so succinctly the *zeitgeist* of mid-century medical modernism (Spellberg and Taylor-Blake, 2013; Specter, 2015). This shared mood was not limited to physicians, either: as historian Nancy Tomes reminds us, a 'gospel of germs' which promised a modern lifestyle free from infectious disease if one only purchased the proper brand-name goods swiftly became a mainstay of American consumer culture over the course of the twentieth century (Tomes, 1998; 2006).

At the extreme end of that promise was the sweeping vision of eradication: irreversibly erasing a scourge of humanity through aggressively disease-focused public health plans that linked prophylactic and therapeutic technologies with martial order. While some form of eradication ideal can be dated back to the Enlightenment, its modern form took on special importance in the American brand of tropical medicine. This field was born in local campaigns against cholera and yellow fever in militarized spaces of American-occupied Havana and Panama by military medics Walter Reed and William Gorgas, then applied more broadly in hookworm eradication campaigns in the American South and, later, the global South in an expansive set of campaigns funded by the Rockefeller Foundation – that likewise propelled the Rockefeller Foundation into the largest single funder of international health programmes in the first half of the twentieth century (Espinosa, 2009; Ettling, 1982; Cueto, 1995; Birn and Solórzano, 1997; Palmer, 2010).

The career of Fred Soper (1893–1977) helps to connect the dream and the reality of 'vertical' or centralized disease-focused public health efforts in international health (Stepan, 2011; Packard, 2007; 2016). Soper cut his teeth on 1930s–40s yellow fever eradication campaigns in South America for the Rockefeller Foundation and the Pan American Health Organization, and emerged in the 1950s to become a central organizing figure in the World Health Organization's sprawling, expensive and ultimately disastrous efforts to eradicate malaria in the second half of the twentieth century. Historian Nancy Stepan has characterized Soper as 'a man absolutely possessed by what he believed was a radical, even revolutionary idea – the idea of the possibility of the complete eradication of disease' (Stepan, 2011, 13). Yet by the time of Soper's death in 1977, this goal of absolute zero had not come to pass in hookworm, yellow fever or malaria. And even though Soper's eradicationist philosophy would be posthumously vindicated three years later when the cover of *World Health* magazine proudly announced that 'Smallpox is Dead!', that success has also been limited: no other human disease has been eradicated since.[3]

Nonetheless, the alert reader will notice that malaria is no longer endemic to the United States, nor to Italy, Bulgaria, Hungary or Romania, nor Australia, nor Cuba or Singapore or Jamaica, Puerto Rico or Taiwan. Yellow fever, diphtheria, polio and many other diseases once common in port cities in North

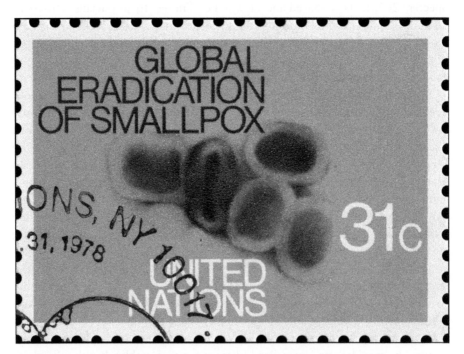

FIGURE 3.1: United Nations Global Eradiation of Small Pox Stamp, 1978. Credit: Dragan Ilic / Alamy Stock Photo.

America and Western Europe are now only endemic elsewhere. Yet all countries in sub-Saharan Africa that now have endemic malaria were, paradoxically, excluded from the initial strategy of the Global Malaria Eradication Program (Webb, 2014; Litsios, 2015). In other words, where eradication has been locally successful, a patchwork of national and regional public health efforts, along with differential economic and political development, has effectively shifted the burden of this disease *elsewhere*: a geography of displacement rather than universal eradication. Over the course of the twentieth century, many have mapped this displacement of the burden of infectious disease: retreat of from the more developed economies of the global North, to a concentrated belt of infectious disease morbidity and mortality in the less developed economies of the global South (King 2003a; 2003b).

The consequences of this displacement soon preoccupied physicians and public health concerns in both developed and developing countries. Although, as historian George Weisz has shown, the meanings of 'chronic disease' were sketched very differently in the US compared to the UK or France or Germany, it was evident to many observers in Europe and North America that overall mortality from epidemic infectious disease had declined remarkably by the middle decades of the twentieth century, while the mortality rates of 'modern epidemics' from noninfectious sources – chief among them cancer, heart disease and stroke – had grown apace (Jones and Greene, 2013). Many warned of a mismatch between a public health system based on hospitals and acute care treatments increasingly out of sync with the epidemiology of disease and death in North America.

In this environment, calls to bolster societal investment in basic research, epidemiology, treatment and prevention of chronic noninfectious diseases found broad institutional support. In Washington, DC, the Albert and Mary Lasker Foundation demonstrated a substantial impact in mobilizing political, financial and scientific support for the construction of new public centres, including the expansion of the singular National Institute of Health into a plural National Institutes of Health, with the foundation of a National Cancer Institute, a National Heart, Lung, and Blood Institute, followed by many more to come, and the launch of the Nixon Administration's ill-fated 'War on Cancer' in 1971 (Patterson, 1989; Davis, 2007).

As the leading causes of mortality shifted from tuberculosis, pneumonia and diarrheal diseases to cancer, stroke and heart disease in the United States and the United Kingdom, many began to refer to these new scourges as 'lifestyle diseases' or 'diseases of civilization'. The idea that the presence of a particular diagnosis could denote a form of societal evolution progress was not new to the twentieth century – witness, for example, George Beard's description of 'neurasthenia' as a uniquely modern malady, which initially chiefly afflicted Americans (Rosenberg, 1977; Stage, 1979). By the early decades of the twentieth century, the increasing visibility of morbidity and mortality from chronic disease like cancer and heart disease within the United State were explicitly understood as a cost of the civilizing process – in a calculus that rendered the diagnosis of these diseases all but invisible in African-American and American Indian populations.[4] Colonial interventions by European and American powers were justified on the basis that hygienic modernity would reduce the infectious disease profile of more, primitive, colonized peoples (Anderson, 2006; Rogaski, 2004; Espinosa, 2009). After the Second World War, the relative burden of acute or chronic disease took on added importance in a newly postcolonial world order in which a new logic of 'developed' and 'developing' worlds was displacing prior imperial distinctions of colonists and colonized. By the late 1960s, modernization theorists at the World Bank and elsewhere began to shift their metrics of development from gross domestic product to more subtle indices of health and well-being (Cruickshank, 2011).

One particularly well-cited model of health and modernity was the epidemiological transition theory of Egyptian-born demographer Abdel Omran.[5] Using the health statistics of the US and UK as an epidemiological goal of development, Omran posited a variant of modernization theory that placed the disease profile of a given society at the centre of an evolutionary narrative from a first 'age of pestilence and famine' to a second 'age of receding pandemics' to arrive at a third and final 'age of degenerative and man-made disease'.

While Omran praised some countries, like Japan, for passing from stage 1 to stage 3 in an 'accelerated transition' through rapid Westernization, he singled out other countries of the developing world – such as Ceylon – as being locked in a 'delayed model' of underdevelopment (Omran, 1971, 522).[6] By the 1980s, a fourth stage, the 'age of delayed degenerative diseases' had been optimistically added to the sequence, noting, for example, the falling rates of morbidity and mortality from coronary artery disease in the United States (Olshansky and Ault, 1986). As Omran's theory of epidemiological transition was swiftly adopted throughout development organizations – often not for the original reasons he advocated – it added the granularity of disease to other metrics of health and development which had focused chiefly on demographic measures of birth and death (Weisz and Olszynko-Gryn, 2010).

As the burden of disease became an increasingly important indicator for economic development towards the close of the twentieth century, international organizations from the World Bank to the World Health Organizations worked to build more and more precise metrics tor measuring them. The 1993 publication of *Investing in Health* by the World Bank signalled the multilateral development organ's intention to jump into the growing field of global health, and set off a series of powerful debates over measurement of the toll any given disease took on a given population. Several metrics – including Quality Adjusted

Life-Years (QALYs) and Disability Adjusted Life-Years (DALYs) – competed to become the universal currency for comparing the impact that diseases from cancer to cholera, diarrhoea to depression took on the economic growth of developing and developed countries alike. Christopher Murray, one of the key architects behind the World Bank report, used these metrics to produce a snapshot of the 'global burden of disease', first used retrospectively to take a high-resolution snapshot of disease around the world in 1990, then prospectively to produce an even more sensitive analytic for 2000, then 2010, then 2015 (Salomon and Murray, 2002; Murray, 2015).

These reports contained some cheering news. Some industrialized nations had indeed entered a 'fourth stage' of the epidemiological transition (such as France, for example, where DALY figures for ischemic heart disease, for example, fell by more than 30% between 1990 and 2013), while other nations, like Mexico, Chile, and Tunisia, had successfully transitioned from the disease burden expected of 'developing' countries towards a more 'developed' disease profile.

But Murray's data also yielded more troubling results. First, in countries in the global North, new infectious diseases had made a mounting comeback: new scourges like HIV/AIDS and antibiotic-immune superbugs from multiple-drug-resistant tuberculosis (MDRTB) to methicillin-resistant *Staphylococcus aureus* (MRSA). As historian Scott Podolsky has pointed out, where once infectious disease specialists feared that the relevance of their own specialty was receding with the advent of broad-spectrum antibiotics, the end of the twentieth century had produced a new post-apocalyptic vision of 'bad bugs, no drugs' (Podolsky, 2014; Infectious Diseases Society of America, 2004). From Richard Preston's *The Hot Zone* to Laurie Garrett's *The Coming Plague*, the turn of the twenty-first century was suffused with increasingly precise predictions of new pandemics to come – a very different moment than what hopeful modernists like Amory Winslow were predicting in the 1940s (Caduff, 2015; Preston, 1994; Garrett, 1994). Well before SARS-CoV-2 shut down the global economy, overturned the rhythms of everyday life, and laid low millions of people around the world in the process, it had become clear that any declaration of the end of the "Age of Epidemics" had been premature.

Second, it has become clear that epidemiological profiles in developing nations have not progressing along a straight line from infectious to chronic disease, recapitulating the North American and European teleology of epidemiological stages. In the face of the HIV/AIDS pandemic, staggering debt to development organs like the World Bank and IMF, and austerity policies gutting public health infrastructures, some countries like Zimbabwe have seen dramatic increases in DALYs attributable to infectious disease. Indeed, by the close of the twentieth century it had become increasingly clear that many countries were now facing the compounded impact of high morbidity from both, as the impact from older scourges like yellow fever, malaria and tuberculosis were joined with modern plagues like Ebola and Zika, on the one hand, and increasing rates of chronic, noncommunicable diseases on the other. In India, Rwanda and many other locations, rising rates of heart disease, cancer and stroke have been tied to the global spread of Western commodities like processed foods and cigarettes (World Health Report, 1999; Boutayeb, 2006; Bygbjerg, 2012; Brandt, 2007). Moreover, infectious diseases like tuberculosis and noninfectious disease like diabetes can interact in especially deadly fashion (Dooley and Chaisson, 2009). The results of this 'double burden of disease' have further complicated any simple modernist tales that the twentieth century was about eradicating disease or even displacing one primitive set of diseases for another, more modern set.

Iterative attempts to map the global burden of disease have also revealed a global burden of mental health afflictions far more extensive than previously acknowledged, and increasing in both scale and scope (Desjarlais et al., 1996). Even though schizophrenia and major mood disorders have stable prevalence across locations and account for a substantial amount of mortality, the public health investment in infrastructures to address mental illnesses has been anaemic at best (Patel, 2003). Many countries have only a handful of trained mental health specialists: India, for example, has one psychiatrist per 200,000–300,000 people, while as of 2012 there was only one psychiatrist to service the roughly 6 million population of Sierra Leone (McDougall, 2012).[7] Calls to rectify this gap rely on metrics like the DALY and QALY to emphasize that the tolls of mental illness are every bit as concrete as those of tuberculosis, heart disease or diabetes. Yet such efforts often run up against the culturally bound specificity with which mental illness categories – beyond the 'big three' of schizophrenia, depression and bipolar disorder – are defined differently in different social contexts.

Recent attempts to rectify the differences between the lists of mental health disorders in the United States (as codified in the *Diagnostic Standard Manual*, 5th edition, or *DSM-V*) and the World Health Organization (as codified in the *International Classification of Disease*, 11th edition, or ICD-11) have yet to produce a universal lexicon of mental health disorders (Jablensky, 2009). Some have criticized the growing application of 'American' mental health diagnoses in surveillance and treatment programmes around the world as a false globalization of disease, a larger marketing ploy on the part of American psychiatrists and pharmaceutical firms (Watters, 2010). The growing burden of mental health disorders raises a familiar question in measuring the overall burden of disease: is the overall rate of depression in the world growing? Are we doing a better job at surveillance? Or have our definitions of disease themselves been changing over time to encompass a broader and broader pool of people?

THE MOBILE DEFINITION OF DISEASE

In spite of general promises to eradicate all infectious diseases, and more specific promises to eradicate a specific subset of infectious diseases, to date Western medicine has intentionally eradicated only smallpox.[8] In the meantime, we have produced lists of diseases that grow with each iteration. The 1869 *Nomenclature of Diseases* drawn up by the Royal College of Physicians enumerated exactly 1,146 diseases, one after another (number 1146, one of three 'injuries not classified', being the ominous 'foreign substances in the cellular tissue') (Royal College of Physicians, 1869, 213). When the ninth version of the World Health Organization's International Classification of Diseases (ICD-9) was ratified just over a century later in 1975, it contained roughly 13,000 entries. Only fifteen years later, when the next iteration (ICD-10) was ratified by the World Health Assembly, the number of diagnoses had increased the number fivefold again to roughly 68,000.

The bureaucratic tasks of implementing these taxonomic changes are enormous. The ICD-10, though ratified by the World Health Organization in 1990, did not see widespread uptake in American medical practice until 2015. Even at this late date the implementation provoked resistance and ridicule, as health care providers chafed at the absurd level of specificity reflected in codes like W56.22 ('struck by orca, initial encounter'), V00.01 ('pedestrian on foot injured in collision with roller-skater'), V91.07 ('burn due to water skis on fire'), Z63.1 ('problems in relationship with in-laws') or the occupational hazard of all historians, Y92.241 ('hurt at the library'). Not content to rest on these laurels, the World Health Organization has been working hard on the next iteration, ICD-11, which is anticipated to be approved in 2018 (Martin, 2015).

Why? What forces compel such absurd specificity in diagnosis? As Faber indicated in his *Nosography*, an arc can be traced from the seventeenth to the twentieth centuries by which professional and popular definitions increasingly shifted from a physiological mode – in which every sick individual was sick in their own way – to a more specific mode, in which every disease was a discrete entity, countable, describable, sortable, hung on a taxonomic tree with its close and distant relations in the family of ailments.[9] The medical historian Owsei Temkin would later expand on this distinction between 'physiological' and 'ontological' approaches to disease as a form of dialectic that runs through the course of human history (Temkin, 1977). The ancient Greeks also knew some diseases as ontological, discrete entities, and physiological explanations of disease persist today in fields of psychiatry, endocrinology and oncology – and, I might add, in the current enthusiasm for personalized or precision medicine. But the course of the twentieth century saw ontological conceptions of disease become more and more commonplace in professional and popular realms across Europe, North America and much of the rest of the world.

Some scholars, following Michel Foucault's 1963 analysis in *Naissance de la clinique*, have looked for a decisive moment of rupture when disease became abstractable from the individual foibles of individual bodies into a physical lesion rendered knowable by universal laws of pathological sciences. In Foucault's analysis, this rupture can be traced to a medical revolution that took place in the hospitals of Paris concomitant to the broader revolution in French society. Others, including Foucault's contemporary, the Swiss-American historian Erwin Ackerknecht, emphasize the broader continuity of thought and practice that link the physicians of the 'Paris Clinic' with earlier and later attempts to characterize disease as a specific and localizable lesion. If Marie François Xavier Bichat (1771–1802) and his followers in Paris characterized the location of specific *morbid tissue* as the seat of disease, they borrowed from earlier physicians like Giovanni Battista Morgagni (1682–1771) who had earlier postulated the affected organ as the seat of disease, and would be leaned on in turn by later pathologists, such as Rudolf Ludwig Carl Virchow (1821–1902) in characterizing disease on the level of the cellular and subcellular structures.

From organ to tissue to cell, the progress of the pathological gaze in eighteenth- and nineteenth-century Europe is often characterized in terms of shrinking lesions, the power of reductionism, the increasing specificity of scientific analysis to sort further the taxonomy of human ailments with finer and finer brushstrokes. As the philosopher Edmund Pellegrino noted in the late 1970s, no small part of the increasing power of diagnostic and therapeutic claims came from the ability to reduce disease to corpuscular mechanisms that functioned on smaller and smaller fields of action (Pellegrino, 1979). Witness, for example, the movement to molecular and genetic medicine after the British physician Archibald Garrod described a child who came to his clinic with black diarrhoea as having a chemical disease, 'alkaptonuria', which he could characterize by 1902 as an inherited molecular 'inborn error of metabolism' (Garrod, 1902). Likewise the 1949 announcement by physical chemist Linus Pauling, that sickle-cell anaemia could be explained on the basis of a genetically determined variant – a single amino-acid – in the molecular structure of haemoglobin allowed Pauling to announce that he had discovered the 'first molecular disease' (Wailoo, 2001, 4–5).

Over the course of the twentieth century, the turn to molecular explanations of disease had offered some increasingly powerful interventions. One thinks of the advent of diagnostic blood tests for syphilis, pregnancy, HIV/AIDS and Ebola, let along the promise of new disease-specific genetic tests from Huntington's disease to breast cancer. So, too, has the molecular turn provided powerful therapeutic tools, from beta-blockers to statins, to proton-pump inhibitors, to selective serotonin reuptake inhibitors and anti-retrovirals, which have all enabled life-saving therapies based on the characterization of molecular pathways. But the shrinking of the biomedical field of action also had the rather unsettling effect of chopping up the sick person into a series of treatable parts rather than a whole person.

Writing in 1970, the British sociologist Nicholas Jewson contrasted the early modern understanding of the sick man as a 'conscious human totality', with the fragmentation of the patient by the late twentieth century into 'a collection of synchronized organs, each with a specialized function', and asked what was lost in that transaction (Jewson, 1970). Many others, including the itinerant philosopher-theologian Ivan Illich, questioned the benefit of a biomedical science that objectified everything it encountered in the name of science without necessarily providing subjectively or objectively better care for the patient (Illich, 1974a). By the early 1980s, these critiques of biomedical reductionism could be found across multiple fields of the social sciences. Sociologists like Renee Fox warned of the dehumanizing basis of the objectifying medical gaze (Fox, 1979). Medical anthropologists such as Arthur Kleinman and Leon Eisenberg depicted biomedical reductionism as a wedge engendering a widening schism between the patient's experience of illness and the objectified category of disease (Kleinman, 1980; Eisenberg and Kleinman, 1981). Historians like Allan Brandt likewise argued that for all its power, biomedical reductionism provided 'no magic bullet' against patterns of disease epidemiology that were rooted in social marginalization and stigma, such as sexually transmitted diseases, sickle-cell anaemia and the newly described AIDS (Brandt, 1985; Wailoo, 2000).

These critiques were also visible from within the world of biomedical science, which had for centuries worked to produce its own antireductionisms and holisms (Harrington, 1996; Debru, 2002). As Barton Childs, the evangelist of genetic medicine at Johns Hopkins, spelled out his 1999 volume *Genetics: The Logic of Disease*,[10] a balance between the 'Oslerian medicine' that sees the body as a generic 'broken machine' and 'Garrodian medicine' that sees each body as unique form of 'chemical individuality' would be necessary to practise medicine on both molecular and human scales. By 2010, as editors at *Scientific American* among others asked why the Human Genome Project had 'failed so far to produce the medical miracles that scientists promised' (Hall, 2010), a nascent field of systems medicines sought new ways to put the patient back together again. Likewise, as a key article in the *Journal of the American Medicine* noted in 2009, new sciences of 'personalized medicine' could use 'connectivity and integration and multiple levels of systems medicine – extending medicine beyond reductionism' (Federoff and Gostin, 2009). In turn, the recent rise of a field of 'network medicine', which draws from mathematical graph theory on the one hand, and the sociology of networks on the other, attempts to map the understanding of disease as a complex interactive field, not reducible to a single mechanism or lesion (Loscalzo et al., 2017).

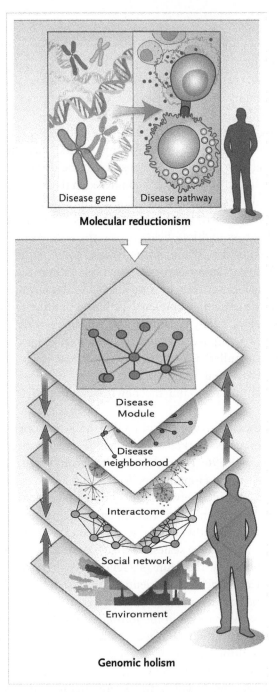

FIGURE 3.2: From Jeremy A Greene and Joseph E. Loscalzo, "Putting the Patient Back Together Again: Social Medicine, Network Medicine, and the Limits of Reductionism," *New England Journal of Medicine* 2017; 377: 2493-2499. Credit: Massachusetts Medical Society, 2017.

These criticisms from both outside and inside of biomedical science and practice increasingly problematize the bestiary of objects collected inside of twentieth- and twenty-first-centuries lists of diseases. On the one hand, the increasing girth of the *ICD-11* or the *DSM-5* could be read as a sign that our descriptions of disease are simply becoming more precise, captured with degree of resolution that can parse each individual twiglet rather than merely the bigger and smaller branches, and consequently occupying a larger data file. Yet the overall utility of this project of parsing smaller and smaller itself is now increasingly questioned, as are its unintended consequences.

PORTRAIT OF A DISEASE IN MOTION: DIABETES

If there are problems in parsing each twig in the taxonomy of disease, it is equally difficult to grasp the structure of the entire tree. In order to illustrate better the processes by which definitions of disease have changed over time – and the consequences of those changes – it might be first approach a single, sturdy branch in the tree of diseases, and witness its growth and contortions over the twentieth and twenty-first centuries. There are so many to choose from—syphilis, depression, the common cold, influenza, heart disease, cancer – and each would trace a different story. But for now I would like to call on a particularly paradigmatic chronic disease: diabetes.

In early 2016, the United States government announced a new programme for Medicare to fight the disease of diabetes by preventing it outright. As Sylvia Mathews Burwell, the Secretary of Health and Human Services, announced in a press conference in New York City, this application of the 2010 Affordable Care Act would pay for 'lifestyle change programs' to coach Americans on healthier eating habits and improved physical activity to prevent the onset of type II diabetes. These programmes had been proven effective in the 86 million American adults estimated to have a condition called 'prediabetes' (Pear, 2016).

To many Americans, prediabetes was a new disease, or at least a new predisease: an abnormality of carbohydrate metabolism that caused circulating blood sugars to be higher than normal, but not quite as high as the pathological state of diabetes. This was a condition of risk: people with prediabetes died more often of strokes and heart attacks; they were more likely to progress to the frank disease of diabetes. This condition might not be worth treating with prescription drugs, perhaps, but it was worth screening, identifying, and addressing with exercise and diet (Knowler et al., 2002).

And yet the condition of prediabetes was not new, nor was the idea of screening for it: the concept had been articulated some seventy-five years earlier, for example, by Charles Best (who, along with Frederick Banting, shared credit and Nobel Prize money for discovery of insulin) when he gave the keynote address at the first annual meeting of the American Diabetes Association in 1941. 'One of the great problems for clinicians and experimentalists,' Best argued, 'is to attempt, perhaps by entirely new means, a way to detect the patients who are on the verge of diabetes' (Best, 1963). Best was only one voice among many in the mid-twentieth century arguing that the group of people at risk for diabetes – called many names, including protodiabetics, chemical diabetics, latent diabetics, stress diabetics and prediabetics – should be identified and treated prophylactically to prevent the debilitating disease.

Yet if one reads closely into these earlier definitions of prediabetes, one finds a curious relation of disease, predisease and history. Take, for example, the 1939 claim by University of Michigan endocrinologist Jerome Conn, that prediabetes involved a measurable abnormality in blood sugars without the telltale sign of sugar in the urine (or glycosuria) that defined the disease of diabetes itself (Newburgh and Conn, 1939). Conn and Banting were arguing, in the middle of the twentieth century, that the disease of diabetes – knowable through urine tests – could be prevented by a screening effort that measured people's blood sugars and targeted populations with abnormally high blood sugars. The CDC's screening guidelines in the early twenty-first century, in contrast, suggest that the disease of diabetes – knowable through blood tests – could be prevented by a screening effort that simply lowered the threshold for action.

What is going on here? How can it be that what was 'prediabetes' in 1941 has simply become 'diabetes' by 2016? The history of diabetes opens a window into the dynamism of disease categories over time, and suggests different ways that historical analysis can provide insights into fundamental problems of diagnosis, therapeutics and the contingent nature of disease itself. These changes don't neatly fit into a progressive narrative of cure and eradication of an otherwise stable disease. Rather, moments like the discovery of insulin, or the development of a screening test for blood sugar, become events that themselves take part in reshaping the aetiology and epidemiology of diabetes itself.

Instead of shrinking, the problem of diabetes has grown in scope and in scale with each of these advances, increasing dramatically in both incidence and prevalence in the ninety years since the introduction of insulin (Centers for Disease Control and Prevention, 2014).[11] To the historian, then, diabetes is a persistent problem, on the one hand knowable (like cancer, or many other chronic diseases) for centuries if not millennia, yet on the other hand constantly changing in form and definition. Is the rising diabetes epidemic of the early twenty-first century the result of changing social determinants – including diet, physical activity and obesity? Or is it the product of a changing definition of what counts as diabetes?

Over time, diabetes has broadly shifted from a condition described chiefly in terms of symptoms felt by the patient to a disease chiefly described in terms of signs visible to the trained eye of the physician, and then into a condition chiefly described in terms of numbers and thresholds set by committees. Some version of diabetes as a symptomatic disease can be found described in the Ebers Papyrus some 3,500 years ago, though not given the Greek name diabetes (the Greek term for 'siphon', a reference to the most common symptom, copious urination) until the first century AD by Arataeus of Cappadocia. A collection of ancient writings from the Egyptian, Greek and Roman corpus nonetheless all coincides on a classical tetrad of symptoms: polyuria (frequent urination), polydipsia (frequent thirst), polyphagia (frequent hunger) and autophagia (wasting) describing a serious disease with poor prognosis.

This overwhelmingly symptomatic basis for defining diabetes shifted, however, with increasing attention to the characteristics of the urine. Although the medieval Persian physician Avicenna had mentioned the honey-like sweetness of diabetic urine, it was not until the seventeenth century that Oxford physician Thomas Willis distinguished the characteristic taste of the urine in diabetes mellitus (adding the Latin word for honey to the Greek word for siphon) and suggested that astute physicians would notice that the urine was 'wonderfully sweet, like sugar or honey'. By the eighteenth century, another English physician, Matthew Dobson, demonstrated that sugar could be detected in the urine of diabetic patients using a relatively simple chemical procedure. In the nineteenth and the early twentieth century, the formal diagnosis of diabetes rested on obtaining urine, acidifying it in a test tube and heating that test tube over a flame to test for the presence or absence of sugar. The normal body produced no sugar in its urine; the diabetic one did.

This shift in the level of diagnosis in the eighteenth and nineteenth centuries – from a discussion of *symptoms* felt by the patient but interpreted by the doctor towards an elucidation of *signs* that were invisible to the patient but could be elucidated from the body of the patient by the trained eye of the physician (increasingly with the help of laboratory equipment) is followed by an equally important shift in the twentieth century: diagnosis by *number*. Already by the nineteenth century a number of clinicians and scientists had noticed that the presence of sugar in the urine was also matched by a high level of sugar in diabetic blood. Yet the mere presence of sugar in the blood couldn't simply be seen as an indication of disease like sugar in the urine could. As the French physiologist Claude Bernard noted, some level of sugar (or glycaemia) was always found in the blood of all vertebrates – indeed the absence of sugar was incompatible with life. Rather, in diabetes, one found that the level of sugar in the blood passed over a threshold – like the water level of a river rising over a dam – that suddenly caused it to spill over into the urine itself.

This vision of diabetes as a disease that could be diagnosed as an abnormally high level of sugar in the blood – before it manifested itself in the pathological sign of sugar in the urine, before in manifested itself in the classical symptoms of polydipsia, polyuria, polyphagia and autophagia – required a different logic

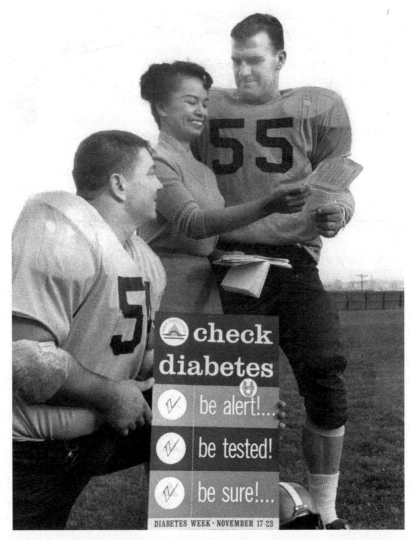

FIGURE 3.3: Dottie Sparlin, staff member of the Mile High United Fund, issues diabetes self detection dreypaks to members of the Denver Broncos squad, Wahoo McDaniel (left) and Jim Fraser. The Colorado Diabetes Association is alerting people to the symptoms and treatment of diabetes. November 16, 1963. Credit: The Denver Post / Contributor / Getty Images.

of diagnosis: setting a numerical threshold for the distinction between the normal and the pathological. At what precise number did the amount of sugar in your blood become a disease? The determination of a single threshold – 126 mg/dL in fasting blood – required more than a physician with chemical reagents: it required the consensus of a committee and the articulation of the late twentieth-century phenomenon of clinical guidelines, which themselves could prove to be highly mobile over time.

Over the late twentieth and early twenty-first centuries, many parties beyond doctor and patient have become interested in these guidelines and their development. The pharmaceutical firm Upjohn, for example, which launched a series of oral diabetic drugs between the 1950s and 1980s, invested heavily in research into prediabetes and sponsored a series of efforts to reshape Conn and Best's categories of prediabetes into the broader category of diabetes, potentially growing the market of consumers of their medications in the process. Upjohn also supported efforts by groups like the American Diabetes Association to expand screening programmes to find the 'million hidden diabetics' in the United States who had a form of diabetes or prediabetes but were unaware of their condition. These partnerships were successful – certainly for Upjohn, whose first oral antidiabetic drug Orinase became an early blockbuster drug, especially in the treatment of these new 'mild diabetics' who would not have been considered diabetics fifty years earlier. These expansions of treatment into what we might call the suburbs of disease left a complex legacy. While they helped, broadly speaking, in the fight against diabetes, they also paradoxically increased the number of people living with diabetes.

It may be worth pausing here for a moment to introduce a few terms introduced by the paediatrician and historian Chris Feudtner, who uses the concept of the 'transmutation of disease' to understand diabetes as a disease in motion (Feudtner, 1996). It should be evident by now that the diagnosis of diabetes has been and continues to be a highly dynamic subject. But Feudtner's concept of 'transmutation' offers an opportunity to look at the role of therapeutics in the transformation of disease as well.

The 1921 discovery of insulin by Macleod, Collins, Banting and Best is typically narrated as a heroic moment in the development of modern biomedicine: the triumph of the laboratory over an ancient scourge (Bliss, 1983). Indeed, the results were dramatic – producing Lazarus-like revivals of children who appeared to be slated for an early and inevitable death. The introduction of insulin extended the lifespan of those afflicted with childhood diabetes by decades upon decades, and this 'wonder drug' has since become an essential medication for millions of people living with diabetes around the world. Yet insulin did not cure diabetes, it did not eradicate it; instead it paradoxically increased rather than decreased the number of people living with the disease. Children with diabetes did not succumb to the condition as children; rather they lived longer lives often to succumb to later, previously unknown manifestations of the disease – conditions like diabetic nephropathy, diabetic neuropathy, diabetic retinopathy and cardiovascular manifestations of diabetes, which became visible as diabetic children grew into diabetic adults. The drug, paradoxically, helped to produce new manifestations of disease, new ways of living and dying with diabetes.

Along with the greater possibility to control the disease came increased moral responsibility for its outcomes. Feudtner uses a remarkable collection of patient materials collected around the early twentieth-century clinic of the Boston-based diabetes specialist Elliot Joslin to describe the changing experience of being a diabetic patient before and after the introduction of insulin (Feudtner, 2003). Insulin therapy was hard work – not merely the mechanical skill of learning to inject oneself safely with insulin by hypodermic syringe, but also the conceptual work of calculating carbohydrate load, the technical work of testing one's own urine for sugar in a makeshift kitchen or bathroom laboratory, and the logistical work of structuring one's life around regular access to all of the materials necessary to manage insulin therapy, day by day, week by week, month by month. Joslin began to give out medals to those patients who maintained good control of their diabetes over several years, and in the case of later medals given by the Joslin Clinic, 'for prolonging life's span after the onset of diabetes, a scientific and moral victory'.

Yet the flip side of the moral victory of successfully managing one's diabetes is the moral responsibility, and blame, that increasingly comes with failure. One unanticipated consequence of the introduction of insulin into diabetes was to help transform the social meanings of a bad outcome from a pitiable affliction into a moral failing. By making diabetes more manageable, insulin also altered the moral discourse of the disease: the patient's own behaviour in complying or not complying with their treatment regimen – not fate, not their genetics – would increasingly be held responsible for their own ill health. In American society, as Arlene Tuchman, Matthew Klingle and Richard Mizelle have recently shown, diabetes was iteratively racialized as it was associated with a series of marginalized populations – Eastern European Jewish immigrants, African-Americans after the Great Migration, American Indians on the reservation, who could be blamed for their high rates of diabetes as a symptom of rapid and incomplete assimilation into modern American life (Tuchman, 2011; Klingle, n.d; Mizelle, 2017). This casual racialization of disease has repeatedly offered a much easier path of blaming disease burden on individual behavior instead of engaging with the structural forces of racism, dispossession, and settler colonialism and their role in producing the stark disparities in health that characterize the modern world.

Similar broad transformations in the social meanings of disease can be found following the introduction of other drugs and medical devices for the management of diabetes. The hypodermic syringe, for example, a symbol of precision in biomedical therapeutics when first introduced in the nineteenth century, had by the mid-twentieth century been broadly associated with an artefact of an underclass of illicit drug users. When Upjohn broadly promoted its new drug Orinase as a tool that offered diabetics 'freedom from the needle', the drug's marketing strategy played off of a host of visible stigmas that the older drug, insulin, presented for people living with diabetes. Yet if the stigma of the syringe complicated the treatment of diabetes, the ease of oral medication created its own problems, as more and more people with milder aberrations of blood sugar were put on Orinase. This became especially relevant after the revelation, at the end of the 1960s, that use of this new drug itself was associated with an increased risk of cardiovascular disease, and again in 2007 when another blockbuster oral drug for diabetes – GlaxoSmithKline's Avandia – was associated with causing cardiovascular disease and death.

The career of diabetes in the twentieth century quickly complicates our understandings of continuity and change in the history of disease. On the one hand, we can trace how the boundaries of a symptomatic disease described in ancient texts could be expanded with the introduction, first, of diagnoses through clinical signs mediated by bedside laboratory techniques, and then by broader numerical thresholds for disease mediated by expert committees at greater and greater distances from the bedside. On the other hand, we can see how the disease category expands via a mobile category of 'prediabetes' from the early twentieth century that links earlier and earlier interventions with broader and broader markets of potential patients. So, too, has the disease been iteratively defined in unexpected ways through its treatments, each new treatment changing the experience of living with a disease in ways neither anticipated at the time nor recorded in simple progressive narratives of therapeutic triumph.

THE BROADER POLITICS OF DISEASE

In spite of these changes, the core status of diabetes as a disease has been pretty unproblematic over the course of the twentieth century. Debates have simmered and continue to burn regarding what threshold constitutes the true definition of diabetes, but the statement that 'diabetes is a chronic disease' has been relatively uncontested, even paradigmatic for millennia. For many other conditions however, the status of being a 'real' disease has been more tightly contested over the course of the twentieth and twenty-first centuries. In the decades since 1920, as the definition of diagnostic categories has taken on greater and greater valence in public and private institutions, the role that the medical profession once reserved to itself in adjudicating normality and pathology has been forced open by other societal actors, from pharmaceutical firms to patient advocacy groups to insurance firms and state bureaucracies.

On 15 December 1973, the Board of Trustees of the American Psychiatric Association voted to change the eighty-one-word definition of the Diagnostic and Statistical Manual (DSM-III) to state that homosexuality was no longer to be considered a disease. This change did not happen merely from within. Much of the impetus behind this change came from a broader gay activist movement who targeted the depathologization of homosexuality as a key political issue after the Stonewall riots of 1969 (Bayer, 1981). When the American Psychiatric

Association held its annual meetings in 1970 in the city of San Francisco, the disease status of homosexuality became a flash point, as gay rights activists infiltrated the conference, and broke up several sessions. But actors within the APA were also crucial to the story – such as John Freyer, a member of a clandestine group of gay psychiatrists calling themselves the 'GayPA', who appeared on a panel in the 1972 APA meetings as 'Dr. H. Anonymous' wearing a Richard Nixon mask and arguing for the removal of homosexuality from the DSM.

Yet the heroic account of gay rights activism in the depathologization of homosexuality – in which the status of homosexuality as a disease is seen as a means of oppression – also elides the historical processes by which homosexuality became pathologized in the first place. In many places, for much of the twentieth century, homosexuality was not a disease but a sin, or a crime, even a capital offence. When physicians such as the Austro-German Richard von Krafft-Ebing proposed that homosexuality be redefined as a pathological category, the definition of homosexuality as disease was seen by many liberal reformers as a means of decriminalizing the condition and restoring civil rights to gay men and women (Hansen, 1989). Well into the 1960s, prominent psychiatrists such as Karl Menninger would tie the medicalization of homosexuality to calls for decriminalization (Bayer, 1981, 39).[12]

The demedicalization of homosexuality had profound negative aftereffects on the legitimacy of psychiatric diagnoses in general. Psychiatry had been held in great esteem in American medicine in the decades following the Second World War, and styled itself as a scientifically based field of medicine (Shorter, 1998; Scull, 2016; Lamb, 2014). Yet the fact that an entire disease category could disappear overnight with the stroke of a pen – in the face of pronounced political pressure – added heft to the arguments that psychiatric diagnoses were social categories, not natural categories. When asked whether other categories like fetishism or voyeurism would soon be removed from psychiatric nosology, a key architect of the DSM responded, 'I haven't given much thought to [these problems] and perhaps that is because the voyeurs and the fetishists have not yet organized themselves and forced us to do that.' Likewise the decision helped to fuel a growing antipsychiatry movement, whose principals sought to puncture what Thomas Szasz labelled the *Myth of Mental Illness* (1961)[13] 'Mental illness is a social construction', Peter Sedgwick noted in 1973, shortly after the APA decision, adding that 'there are no illnesses or diseases in nature'; rather, psychiatric diagnoses were labels that transformed deviance into disease through professional sleight of hand (Spitzer, 1973; Bayer, 1981, 190).[14]

As criticisms of the biological or realist basis of disease grew over the course of the late twentieth century, many reached back to the epistemologist and philosopher of biology, Georges Canguilhem, whose 1943 doctoral thesis – conceived in part while serving as a medic in the French Resistance – was published in English in 1966 as *The Normal and the Pathological*. In this exploration of the relationship of physiology and pathology in the nineteenth and twentieth centuries, Canguilhem posits that there never was, is, or will be any pure science of the pathological, and that the relationship between norms and normality is of necessity a dynamic process. For Canguilhem this was true not merely for psychiatric illnesses but of all somatic illness, from diabetes to high blood pressure to anaemia, indeed even to infectious disease. Echoing René Dubòs, Canguilhem pointed out that the mere presence of M. *tuberculosis* in the body was not enough to cause the disease tuberculosis. Any definition of disease therefore had one foot in the social and the other in the biological (Canguilhem, 1989; Dubòs, 1952).

Canguilhem's most famous student, Michel Foucault – the son and grandson of physicians – would lean more heavily on the social basis of this epistemological formulation. In a series of works on power, discipline, medicine, psychiatry and sexuality, Foucault's writings demonstrated to broad audiences that the physician's ability to define the boundaries of disease was one of the subtlest forms by which a society policed its lines of order and deviance.[15] Nor was Foucault the first critic of the excesses of 'medicalization', a field which already contained philosophers and theologians, sociologists, historians and anthropologists,[16] and a broader set of health activists from civil society (Illich, 1974b; Paton, 1974; Conrad, 1975; Fox, 1977). Health feminist analyses criticized the pathologization of childbirth, hysteria and menopause as an overextension of a predominantly male medical gaze (Smith-Rosenberg, 1974; Ehrenreich and English, 1978; Leavitt, 1986). Marxist critics decried medicalization as an extension of capitalist oppression that diverted attention from the underlying social determinants of health (Waitzkin, 1979). Read jointly, the broader critique of medicalization questioned the power of the medical profession to characterize more and more things as diseases and therefore exert professional control over previously nonpathological categories, from sexual preference to shyness to distraction to old age, menopause and pregnancy.

For many parties in the 1970s and early 1980s, the political critique of medicalization went hand in glove with a cultural critique of disease as socially constructed.[17] Like the term medicalization, 'social construction' initiated as a precise term in the field of the sociology of knowledge – first posited by Peter Berger and Thomas Luckmann in their 1966 *The Social Construction of Reality: A Treatise in the Sociology of Knowledge* (Berger and Luckmann, 1966). By the end of the 1970s, the term had been used to describe the social construction of child abuse, epilepsy and menopause; by the early 1980s the term was widely used to contest the reality of any so-called disease (Gelles, 1975; Rothman, 1977; West, 1979; MacPherson, 1981). Social constructivism came in two forms: a weak form, which suggested that more attention needed to be paid to the social (as well as biological) elements that came to define disease, and a strong form, which suggested that the underlying reality of many diseases was itself a myth that had been socially constructed. Though social scientists of medicine continue to emphasize the utility of 'soft' social constructivism, as the term spread into popular critiques it tended to move with 'hard' form: to expose a disease as 'socially constructed' was to argue that it was not in fact 'real' but rather an exercise of power in some form: professional, political or market-oriented.

In a series of essays published in the *New York Review of Books* beginning in 1978, the influential essayist and public intellectual Susan Sontag reflected on her own experience with the diagnosis of breast cancer to argue this conundrum from the other side. If all diseases, from tuberculosis to cancer, took a social toll on the mind in addition to the biological they took on the body of those afflicted, wasn't the 'social construction' of illness merely another burden for the ill to bear, and therefore something to remove if possible? In Sontag's analysis, published in book form as *Illness and Metaphor*, the dread diseases of the nineteenth and twentieth centuries – tuberculosis and cancer, respectively – were made even more dreadful because of the metaphorical significance they were given. 'Nothing is more punitive than to give a disease a meaning,' Sontag concluded, 'that meaning being invariably a moralistic one.' Peel metaphor away from disease, and perhaps those suffering would suffer less.

Sontag would amend her work in 1989 to reflect the sobering new reality of an epidemic (first called the Gay-Related Immunological Disorder, or GRID, before acquiring the name AIDS) that entailed a previously unknown biological entity (first called the lymphadenopathy-associated virus (LAV) and the human-T lymphotropic virus type III (HTLV-III) before acquiring the name HIV) (Sontag, 1989). HIV/AIDS became visible in American society precisely because it tracked alongside a number of morally charged social categories in American life – initially homosexuality, heroin use, haemophilia and Haitian immigration, clustered in an ignominious early CDC report as the '4-H' club. Yes, AIDS was first described as socially constructed, but it also represented something new under the sun in the material realm. Yes, our initial response to AIDS was hindered by the moral and metaphorical residues attached by its initial marginalization to marginal populations, but then again these metaphors were never fully broken. As anthropologist Arthur Kleinman noted in an review of Sontag's work, 'AIDS, like cancer and heart disease and diabetes, is not only an idea: it is cramping pain, the disturbing sounds and difficult-to-take sights and smalls of basic bodily processes gone terribly-awry, the sting and choke of deep despair, especially the isolation and loneliness that come from near-total preoccupation with survival' (Kleinman, 1989). Rather, he argued, it was crucial to have a way to talk about stigma and disease that did not privilege materialism on the one hand or constructivism on the other, but could maintain both within a binocular field of vision: a biosocial approach.

In the case of AIDS, the transformation of metaphors from the stigma of a 'gay scourge' to the confidence of 'living positively' owes much less to the work of benign physician saviours than it does to patients turned activists. Since that time, the story of how AIDS activists in the 1980s and 1990s transformed the diagnosis of AIDS from one of shame, despair, isolation and loneliness to a rallying cry for human rights and human dignity has rightly been celebrated many times and in many forms.[18]

The story is often told like this: a brave band of gay men takes note of the stigma associated with the illness and rejects it, refusing to be hidden and rather demanding attention, finding power in that attention, using their voices, their writing, their art and their bodies to focus the light repeatedly on the Reagan government, on the policies of the FDA, and get a seat at the table for patients in defining the priorities in managing a devastating disease. Much of this was accomplished through moments that turned the previously invisible shockingly visible, such as the action by ACT UP (AIDS Coalition to Unleash Power) on 12 October 1988, which turned the drab Parklawn Office Building in Rockville, Maryland into the stage for a theatrical protest to 'Seize Control of FDA'. Some protestors wore bloodstained doctors' coats, while others staged a 'die-in', lying down with coffins in front of the office building. Signs called out the FDA Commissioner ('Frank Young, you can't hide, we charge you with genocide!') and the federal government in general ('AIDS Doesn't Discriminate – Our Government Does'). Other protestors wore shirts announcing 'Gay and Positive' (Epstein, 1993; Gould, 2009).

Their tactics worked, and the experience of these early AIDS activists has become a playbook for other groups of patients seeking to identify stigmatization and neglect of their own disease conditions and demand different social, political and economic treatment. But this story also created a sense of who a typical AIDS patient was (white, male, gay, educated, middle-class) that obscured the changing face of the epidemic. It would take subsequent forms of activism to acknowledge the differential survival of patients with HIV/AIDS in countries in the global North and South, or its rising heterosexual transmission among women of colour in the United States.

The history of AIDS activism is also related to an earlier generation of breast cancer activists – including Rose Kushner (1929–90) – a journalist and cancer survivor who like Sontag pushed through a wall of silence and stigma surrounding her own diagnosis to create proud and effective social networks based on disease affiliation. Diagnosed in 1974, Kushner resisted not only the disfiguring radical mastectomy which was then the standard of care, but also the decision process that effectively excluded women from understanding and participating in such decisions. Kushner's popular critiques of the isolation and disempowerment of the breast cancer patient helped to gain national and international attention, which was further mobilized by the construction of a telephone hotline (the Breast Cancer Advisory Center), direct confrontation with organizations of oncologists and surgeons, and the inclusion of patient

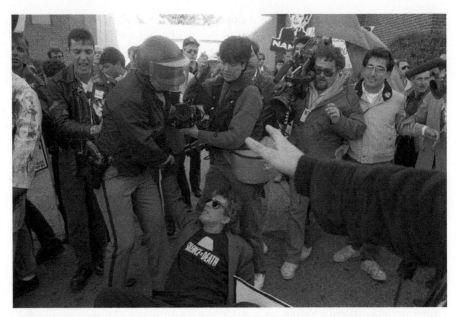

FIGURE 3.4: ACT UP (AIDS Coalition to Unleash Power) at the headquarters of the
Food and Drug Administration (FDA) on October 11, 1988 in Rockville, Maryland.
Credit: Catherine McGann / Contributor / Getty Images.

representatives on NIH panels evaluating treatments for breast cancer (Lerner,
2001; Aronowitz 2007).

Kushner helped to mobilize networks of people united, rather than isolated,
by their diagnoses. Yet as the subsequent development of breast cancer advocacy
has shown, the politics of disease is not merely one of unification. As the
sociologist Maren Klawiter details in her 2008 ethnography *The Biopolitics of
Breast Cancer*, social and political affiliations around the diagnosis have since
fragmented along a number of lines (Klawiter, 2008). The pink ribbon of the
Susan G. Komen Foundation, for example, seems to unify all comers behind its
mission to 'save lives by meeting the most critical needs in our communities and
investing in breakthrough research to prevent and cure breast cancer'. But the
Komen Foundation has come under attack by many breast cancer activists for
its conservative political ideology, its funding threats to reproductive rights
organizations such as Planned Parenthood, its dependence on corporate funding
and its willingness to cross-license the 'pink ribbon' with other brands in
awareness campaigns that some describe as 'pinkwashing'. The latter term was
coined by Breast Cancer Action, a rival breast cancer advocacy group that urges
activists to 'follow the money' and 'think before you pink': to insist on a more
careful critique of corporate involvement in the production of breast cancer

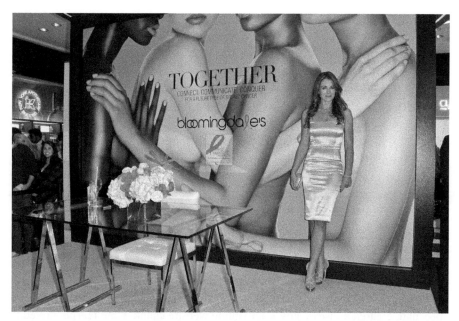

FIGURE 3.5: Elizabeth Hurley attends the Estee Lauder Breast Cancer Awareness
Campaign, Bloomingdale's 59th Street Store on October 20, 2011 in New York City.
Credit: D Dipasupil / Contributor / Getty Images.

through the release of carcinogenic materials in consumer products and the
broader environment.[19]

If HIV/AIDS activism was initially associated with the gay rights movement
in North America, and breast cancer activism with new forms of health feminism,
other forms of disease activism have been associated with alternate civil rights
struggles including race, ethnicity and disability. The early history of sickle-cell
disease activism, for example, has much to do with the haematologists in whose
clinics sickle-cell patients began to cluster. But as the disease came to be associated
with African-American patients, as Keith Wailoo has narrated, the politics of
sickle-cell advocacy quickly became racially inflected, as the social organization
around the disease took shape in a broader social environments: community
organizations, municipal policies and federal entitlements. As with breast cancer,
the realm of sickle-cell advocacy has also fragmented (Wailoo, 2011). The Sickle
Cell Disease Association of America, founded in 1971 as an umbrella organization
for fifteen local advocacy groups, now has extensive corporate partnership and
focuses extensively on genetic counselling, technical training, clinical trials and
new pharmaceutical development. Witness the difference between these aims
and those of the Sickle Cell Warriors, a self-proclaimed online 'judgment free
zone' for sharing experiences with sickle cell disease diagnosis, management,
and its implications for relationships, parenting and careers.

By the close of the twentieth century, breast cancer activism, sickle-cell activism and AIDS activism had become models for other disease-specific advocacy groups, from lupus to ovarian cancer, leukaemia to social anxiety disorder, fibromyalgia to late-stage Lyme disease. The National Alliance on Mental Illness, for example, was founded in 1977 in Madison, Wisconsin, by two parents of children living with schizophrenia; by the 1990s it had become a powerful voice in advocating the destigmatization of psychosis, the rights of schizophrenics in the workplace and public sphere, and the development of new treatments. But in the 1990s, it increasingly came under fire for receiving substantial funding from pharmaceutical corporations and for its support of newer, more expensive antipsychotics – many of which turned out to be no more effective and far less safe than older treatments (Silverstein, 1999).

As pharmaceutical firms learned the benefit of adapting a language of patient empowerment, especially through associations with putatively 'grassroots' organization whose true roots were more artificially woven by their own marketing budgets, the politics of patient advocacy faced an authenticity crisis of co-optation and 'astroturfing'. In 1996, the pharmaceutical firm SmithKline Beecham created a disease advocacy online website called 'Café Herpe' linked to herpes support groups in 'a café-style environment that's fun to use'; the 'Espresso Bar' provided information on Valtrex, SmithKline's new brand-name treatment for the condition, which was much more expensive but no more effective at treating the disease than the generically available drug acyclovir.[20] A year later, SmithKline Beecham helped to found the Social Anxiety Organization, as part of a massive public relations campaign to promoted the disease of Social Anxiety Disorder to lay the groundwork for FDA approval of SKB's product, Paxil, as the sole treatment officially available for the disease (Lane, 2006; 2007).

Tempting as it may be to dismiss this process as manufacturing sickness out of pure cloth, however, or 'selling sickness', it is still true that these bids only work if people buy into them (Moynihan and Cassells, 2006). Socialphobia.org may have been an AstroTurf stadium, but GSK still needed people to come in to occupy the seats, if you will, for it to be worth the expense of construction. Restless Legs Syndrome, one of the newer and more preposterous sounding conditions built around a specific drug (ropinaril) nonetheless has sufferers and their families lined up to testify to the reality of the condition and the great benefit that positive diagnosis and subsequent treatment has brought to their lives. If, in the words of anthropologist Joe Dumit, pharmaceutical marketers are selling us new conditions with our 'surplus health', it is no easy or simple step to point out that the emperor has no clothes (Dumit, 2012). The clothes may happen to be unnecessarily expensive, potentially harmful and wasteful of our resources as individuals and as a society, but they are being worn nonetheless.

In turn, the politics of disease in the early twenty-first century have become a space in which easy dichotomies break down. Patient groups are not necessarily authentic voices of patients protesting the medicalization of physicians – they can be funded by pharmaceutical firms, and at times more invested in medicalization then the doctors themselves.[21] We live in a time in which some gay, bisexual and lesbian communities are working to resist medicalization of sexuality while making arguments based on genetic determinism ('Born This Way'), at the same time that the trans advocacy community is making a social rights case based on an equally vigorous embrace of medicalization (through diagnoses such as gender dysmorphic disorder) that requires a rejection of genetic determinism. The unity of LGBT activism, as with so many forms of identity politics, fractures in the social and biological understandings of disease, and the intense politics involved in navigating that interface.

CONCLUSION

The diagnosis, prognosis and treatment of disease have long been central tasks in the practice of medicine. By the turn of the twentieth century, the sharp delineation of specific disease categories – with the taxonomic structure of the new science of bacteriology as the guide – had become central to the consolidation of new forms of biomedical knowledge and practice. Yet the burden of health and disease, the delineation of normality and pathology, and the kinds of logics used to distinguish them have changed drastically since that time, as both the epidemiology and epistemology of disease continued to transform over the twentieth and twenty-first centuries. In the decades since 1920, as the definition of diagnostic categories has taken on greater and greater valence in public and private institutions, the role that the medical profession once reserved to itself in adjudicating normality and pathology has been forced open by other societal actors, from pharmaceutical firms to patient advocacy groups to insurance firms and state bureaucracies.

How do diseases get defined and demarcated in this wider arena? Who gets to decide what is a disease, and what is not? What are the consequences of such decisions? By the close of the twentieth century, disease could not simply be separated from illness as objective is from subjective, biological is from social. Rather, disease has become an iterative product of politics, bodies, the conceptual and the material worlds, which interact with each other, to transmute disease further, to loop back further on the material and semiotic bases for classifying people as patients (Hacking, 1995).

Knud Faber, compiling his slim and optimistic *Nosography* in 1919, could not have predicted the complexity of the century that was to come: not the increasing burden of chronic maladies, not the resurgence of viral pandemics, not the iterative expansion and incommensurability of the DSM-V and ICD-11, and surely not the scientific, social and political criticism that these trees of diagnoses would produce. Nonetheless, in emphasizing the centrality of the concept of disease in modern medical thought and practice, Faber's work foreshadowed how obsessed we have become with these categories, and how influential they have become as historical actors in their own right: in shifting the burden of morbidity across populations, in defining the legitimacy of individual forms of suffering, and in mapping the broader politics of difference and disparity, rights and entitlements, stigma and social support. The determinants, meanings and responses to disease now constitute a field both biological and social: a vital politics, indeed.

NOTES

1. 'Facebook founder gives $3 billion to end disease' *The Washington Post*, 21 September 2016.
2. 'Taking disease "personally": Columbia University's Precision Medicine Initiative', 10 September 2015. Accessed online at http://columbiaeye.org/about-us/news-and-events/taking-disease-personally-columbia-universitys-precision-medicine.
3. Though a nonhuman disease, rinderpest, has been eradicated since that time, and polio, Chagas' disease and leprosy have also come close – not to mention the mobilized fear of the potential for a return of smallpox in weaponized form.
4. On the inability of physicians to diagnose cancer or heart disease in African-American patients in the first decades of the twentieth century, see Keith Wailoo, *How Cancer Crossed the Color Line*; and Anne Pollock, *Medicating Race; Heart Disease and Durable Preoccupations with Difference*. On the invisibility of chronic disease among American Indians in the first half of the twentieth century, see David S. Jones, *Rationalizing Epidemics: Meanings and Uses of American Indian Mortality Since 1600*.
5. Portions of this section from 'Pharmaceutical Geographies: Mapping the Boundaries of the Therapeutic Revolution'. See also Arturo Escobar, *Encountering Development: The Making and Unmaking of the Third World*; James C. Scott, *Seeing Like a State: How Certain Schemes to Improve the Human Condition Have Failed*; Nils Gilman, *Mandarins of the Future, Modernization Theory in Cold War America*; and Michael Latham, 'Modernization', in Theodore Porter and Dorothy Ross (eds.), *The Modern Social Sciences*.
6. This analysis builds on Paul Cruickshank's account of the convergence of health and the logics of development in the long 1970s. Paul J. Cruickshank, *The Teleology of Care: Reinventing International Health, 1968–1989*.
7. Jeshoor Jebadurai, 'One psychiatrist per 200,000 people', *Royal College of Psychiatrists: Overseas Blogs*, accessed at http://www.rcpsych.ac.uk/discoverpsychiatry/overseasblogs/india/onepsychiatristper200,000.aspx.
8. Technically, two: the world was declared free of the cattle disease rinderpest in 2011. Donald G. McNeil, 'Rinderpest, Scourge of Cattle, is Vanquished', *New York Times*, 27 June 2011.
9. Faber, *Nosography*; Owsei Temkin would later amplify this distinction in a well-cited essay on the distinction between physiological and ontological approaches to disease.

10. This argument initially published as: Barton F. Childs, 'The Logic of Disease', in *The Metabolic and Molecular Basis of Inherited Disease*, 7th edition.

11. Centers for Disease Control and Prevention. National diabetes statistics report: estimates of diabetes and its burden in the United States, 2014. Atlanta, GA: U.S. Department of Health and Human Services, Centers for Disease Control and Prevention, 2014.

12. It should be noted that in the UK, the Wolfendon Report of 1963 called for both decriminalization and depathologization. Menninger's introduction to the American publication of this document agreed with the former but not the latter. Great Britain Committee on Homosexual Offenses and Prostitution, 1963.

13. Thomas Szasz, *The Myth of Mental Illness: Foundations of a Theory of Personal Conduct*. See also D.G. Cooper, *Psychiatry and Anti-Psychiatry*; Thomas Szasz, *The Manufacture of Madness: A Comparative Study of the Inquisition and the Mental Health Movement*; and Allan V. Horwitz, *Creating Mental Illness*.

14. Robert Spitzer, as quoted in the *New York Times*, 23 December 1973, sec 4, p. 5, as cited in Bayer, *Homosexuality and American Psychiatry*, p. 190. See also Howard Becker, *Outsiders*; Erving Goffman, *The Presentation of Self in Everyday Life*; and *Stigma*; Thomas J. Scheff, *Being Mentally Ill*; Edwin M. Schur, *Labeling Deviant Behavior*; Walter R. Gove, *The Labeling of Deviance: Evaluating a Perspective*; and Walter R. Gove (ed.), *Deviance and Mental Illness*.

15. See *The Birth of the Clinic*; *Madness and Civilization*; *Discipline and Punish*, etc.

16. See historians, sociologists, anthropologists of medicalization.

17. For a longer review of social constructivism in the social sciences of medicine, see Ludmilla Jordanova, 'The Social Construction of Medical Knowledge', in John Warner and Frank Huisman (eds.), *Locating Medical History: The Stories and Their Meanings*. Though Jordanova seeks to make the distinction that 'there is no inherent link between 'medicalization' and a social constructionist approach . . . indeed in some ways they are historiographically at odds', nonetheless in popular usage the two have become frequently conflated.

18. E.g. documentary films like Randy Shilts's *And the Band Played On* (1993); popular films from *Philadelphia* (1993) to *The Dallas Buyers' Club* (2013); historical and sociological accounts like Elizabeth Fee and Daniel Fox's *AIDS: The Making of a Chronic Disease*; and Epstein's *Impure Science*.

19. http://thinkbeforeyoupink.org/resources/before-you-buy.

20. 'Café Herpe enters the web', *Advertising Age*, 20 November 1996; 'Café Herpe serves up unappetizing fare: to avoid heartburn, just skip the site', *Advertising Age*, 25 November 1996.

21. Consider, here, the case of end-stage Lyme disease, or DMD drugs approved over the protest of the FDA advisory board.

CHAPTER FOUR

Animals

ROBERT G. W. KIRK

ANIMALS, AND THE ECOLOGICAL VISION OF HEALTH AND WELL-BEING

At the dawn of the twenty-first century, Thomas Thwaites, a London-based 'speculative' designer, felt that his life had become too much of a burden. Thwaites was worried. He was worried about the future. He worried about his prospects. His career. His health. The impact that worrying was having on his health. He worried about the planet's health. Climate change. The collapsing ecosystem and the emerging reality that the world had entered a sixth great extinction. He worried about the widening gap between those with money and those without. He worried about terrorism. The economy. He worried over whether there was a future to worry about and whether that future had a place for him and those he cared about and worried for. His family worried too. So were his friends. Everyone he knew seemed to be worried. Everyone except his niece's dog, Noggin. Animals, it seemed to Thwaites, lacked what now appeared an all too human characteristic: the tendency to worry about the future. Thwaites realized that he needed to escape his worries. He needed a holiday: a holiday from being human. This entailed escaping the constraints and expectations not just of society, culture, personal history and selfhood, but Thwaites's very biology. Thwaites became a goat. Or more properly, in becoming animal, he became something entirely new: a GoatMan (Thwaites, 2016).

For Thwaites, becoming a goat was a therapeutic escape from the stress of being human. Becoming animal was a positive choice to enhance his well-being. A hundred years earlier, in the closing years of the nineteenth century, becoming animal held quite different meanings for H. G. Wells. Far from being a desirable

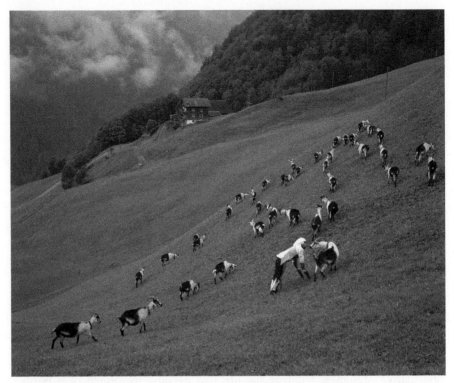

FIGURE 4.1: GoatMan, Thomas Thwaites. Credit: Tim Bowditch.

choice, becoming animal evoked negative connotations: degeneration, the debasement of all that was good in human being, the end of civilization. In *The Island of Doctor Moreau* (1896), Wells presented the eponymous Doctor's geographic isolation from humankind mirrored his moral position as he applied experimental science to create human-like animal hybrids. In what can be read as a thinly veiled critique of 'vivisection', medical science's blurring of the line between human and animal was depicted as a corruption not just of the bodies and behaviours of the biologically altered but also the moral values and ethical judgement of Moreau himself as a human being. One hybrid creature, 'Satyr-man', part human and part goat, evoked the classical image of Satan as cloven hooved and was described in the novel as 'Satanic' (Wells, 1975[1896]: 94). For Wells, becoming animal was likened to becoming not just bestial but the beast itself.

Thwaites' GoatMan and Wells' Satyr-man reveal the long-standing practice of defining and valuing what is human against what is animal. Contrasting the two reveals the essential nature of the 'human' to be culturally situated and thus malleable, which is to say the human is nothing if not historical. Contrasting the two equally invites the question: what changed? How did the twentieth century transform a culture (in this case a male British middle class white culture) from the valorization of the human (and its converse, an antipathy to the animal) to its alternative: a longing to escape the human through actively becoming animal? An adequate response to this question would be beyond the bounds of any short chapter. Instead, our ambition is limited to surveying the role of medical knowledge in questioning the boundaries of the human across the twentieth century. Our conceit is that such questioning modestly contributed to generating active desires to move away from understanding the human as other than animal and towards a much more intimate association of human and animal life.

Such a proposal is radical. Radically positive for some in that it harbours a fluid potential for a fairer future. Radically dangerous for others. Yet if, as Foucault suggests, the '[hu]man is an invention of recent date. And one perhaps nearing its end', then what are we to do with this knowledge? By shoring up a concept soon to be bequeathed to the past, we ensure only that the stories we tell are to eventually fade with the image of the human upon which they are grounded. In contrast, a properly historical response would be to embrace the erosion of the human idol by the seas of cultural change. Only in this way might we hope to produce history of relevance to tomorrow. In recent decades across the humanities, social sciences and life sciences, a shared desire to critique and rethink the prominence of the human within academic narratives has emerged. Yet questioning what it is to be human remains for many a modern-day heresy. Within medical history, Roger Cooter has written forcefully against any attempt 'to place humans on a par with animals, plants, and other nonhuman material things'. He warns not only of a threat to 'writing academic history' but also of 'worrying political implications' (Cooter with Stein, 2013: 10). If we are to believe Cooter, as it would seem some medical historians are all too ready to do, any challenge to humanism inevitably leads to totalitarian politics of the worst form (ibid., 205–28). Such a sweeping claim, collapsing a variety of diverse writings each reaching beyond the human in distinctive ways, is akin to throwing the post-human baby out with the bathwater. Just as there are many shades of humanism there are multiple approaches to rethinking what it is to be human. Of the latter, not all embrace the post-human. Not all place the human on a par with other forms of agency. And not all are apolitical. Indeed, the call to move beyond human-exceptionalism is frequently (albeit problematically) made in the service of preserving the humanities. Fostering a more humble understanding of our human being is presented as a first step toward building a more humane world. By placing Bruno Latour and ANT so firmly in his sight Cooter blinds the history of medicine to theorists of the more than human whose intent and work is both compatible with historical writing *and* arguably more politically aware than what is all too often normative for the discipline. At the risk of attempting to out-Cooter Cooter in taking a provocative stance against his provocation, one might argue that his standpoint not only fundamentally misrepresents the more than human turn (if such that it is) but in doing so firmly anchors the history of medicine to a sinking ship. In contrast, the work of Rosi Braidotti (2012; 2013) and Donna Haraway (e.g. 2003; 2016), to name but two important examples, offers a renewed political agenda which preserves and extends the traditional task of the humanities by rendering critical thinking fit for purpose in a post-disciplinary world.

THE JANUS FACE OF MEDICINE: ONE HEALTH, TWO HEALERS?

In the modern Western era, human medicine and its history became divided from veterinary (which is to say all other animal) medicine. In 1993, Roy Porter lamented 'the sad fact that historians of human medicine and historians of veterinary medicine seem to have relatively little contact with each other' (Porter, 1993: 19). At the same meeting, veterinary epidemiologist Calvin W. Schwabe echoed this view from the perspective of health practitioners. Schwabe called for a greater embrace of the idea of 'one health' which 'had been recognised only intermittently and with varying degrees of comprehensiveness' despite human and veterinary medicine sharing 'virtually identical scientific underpinnings' (Schwabe, 1993). Schwabe, a prominent twentieth-century advocate of a 'one medicine' approach to medicine, illustrates how the notion of health and medicine as transcendent of human-animal boundaries was integral to twentieth-century medicine while being simultaneously concealed (Schwabe, 1964). Proponents of 'one medicine' often cite the nineteenth-century German physician and comparative pathologist Rudolf Virchow, who claimed that 'there is no scientific barrier, nor should there be, between veterinary medicine and human medicine; the experience of one must be utilized for the development of the other' (Saunders, 2000). Virchow contributed to medicine the category of 'zoonosis', having recognized that many infectious diseases are shared across species caring little as to whether their host is human or animal (Wilkinson, 1992). Similarly, William Osler, one of the 'great men' of classic medical history, has been successfully appropriated to the cause having been established (with no credible evidence) as having originated the term 'one medicine'.[1] From the mid-twentieth century, figures such as Virchow and Osler have been rhetorically mobilized in an attempt to make visible the fact that the apparently transgressive idea of 'one medicine' was actually the bedrock of modern scientific medicine (e.g. Schwabe, 1964). While such challenges have in recent years gained ground, overall the division of human and veterinary medicine has remained a powerful social, economic, conceptual and practical boundary.

One consequence of the professional divide between human and veterinary medicine having robustly weathered the challenge of 'one medicine' is that the consequent structural difference has been inherited as a rarely questioned frame for medical history. Accordingly, within conventional histories of epidemiology and public health, two areas where human and animal health are most prominently connected, human medicine is brought to the fore while animals appear merely as the canvas upon which understandings of disease have been mapped, contained and understood (Hardy, 2014). Early ties between medical professional and medical historian, subsequently supported by the investment of both in disciplinary and professional identity as means to legitimacy, have ensured that the history of medicine mirrored its object. For instance, early interest in the history of medicine as a 'profession' produced narratives, which pre-established in their very question the separation of human and veterinary medicine into two 'professions' with separate points of origin and sites of authority. Similarly, historical accounts of medical education in the modern period make little reference to veterinary education (cf. Bonner, 1995; Swabe, 1999). Only in the sphere of public health do the two occasionally coalesce (e.g. Hardy, 2002). In sum, medical history has tended to reinforce rather than challenge the assumed human-exceptionalism that legitimated and made possible the separation of human from veterinary medicine.

Yet history exists in the present, not the past. With the postmodern age has come growing recognition of the integrated almost ecological relationship of human to animal health. From the late twentieth century, in part a result of worlds becoming both singular and smaller in the wake of globalization, 'new' and 'emerging' diseases such as Lassa and COVID-19 not only re-established infectious disease as a major medical concern but also firmly entangled human with animal health (as well as the health of the developed with that of the developing world).[2] Modern 'industrialized' food production, too, demonstrated the entangled nature of the two, as human diseases such as Creutzfeldt–Jakob disease (vCJD or nvCJD) were linked to their animal precursor bovine spongiform encephalopathy (BSE), or 'mad cow disease' (Ridley and Baker, 1998). Continued warnings against the use of hormones and antibiotics within intensified agricultural systems, and more recent concerns about avian and swine flu's capacity to cross species boundaries and trigger potential global pandemics, have all contributed to the recasting of intensive farming practices as critical fault lines generative of both health *and* illness (Cantor et al., 2010). As such, early twenty-first-century medical culture is much more receptive to the notion that disease, particularly infectious disease, can and arguably should be seen as a platform for human and animal medicine; an invitation to integrative understandings of human and animal health. Medical history cannot and has not ignored this trend. But our response has barely begun.

Michael Bresalier, Angela Cassidy and Abigail Woods present an overview of 'one health in medicine', illustrating how modern 'human medicine' has 'a rich history of engagement with animals, their diseases and the people and institutions dedicated to animal health' (Bresalier et al., 2015: 10). They caution against any 'simple, linear narrative linking past to present' and reject arguments such as that of Schwabe by asserting 'direct lessons from history, or to claim – as do many existing histories – that the work of certain historical figures demonstrates the importance of pursuing One Health today'. Nevertheless, history is important in revealing that health is the result of a complexity of interconnections across the human-animal boundary. The interconnectedness of humans, animals and the environment is deeply embedded in medicine across history, shaping (and presumably being shaped by) changing knowledge and practices of health over time. Yet it is unclear what we should take the consequence of this observation to mean. Bresalier et al., for example, highlight the centrality of animals in the development and acceptance of 'germ theory' through reference to cattle plague epidemics (which drew the attention of human medical and veterinary investigators alike) and the work of Louis Pasteur and Robert Koch. At the same time, Bresalier et al. claim, 'germ theory . . . undermined' one health by displacing the prominence of 'environment' in narratives of disease (Bresalier et al., 2015: 6). While the development of 'disease ecology' in the mid-twentieth-century work of Theobald Smith, F. Macfarlane Burnet, René Dubos and Frank Fenner (amongst others) went some way to move bacteriology away from overly reductionist narratives narrowly focused on infectious pathogens to produce what Warwick Anderson (2004) has described as a 'complex, biologically informed epidemiology', clearly the role of animals in the development of concepts such as 'germ theory' is far from straightforward. Bresalier et al. suggest that 'these interconnections can be explained, in part, by reference to prevailing scientific ideas, practices and disease problems, but they can only be fully understood by examining the people involved, their institutional settings and the wider professional, political, economic and environmental contexts' (Bresalier et al., 2015: 10). From this approach, 'germ theory' may well have contributed to the formation of public health concerns that challenged the separation of human from animal health. But professional divisions and competition for money, authority and prestige ensured that (human) medical and veterinary disciplinary differences were structurally embedded within political, educational and cultural institutions (Bresalier et al., 2015: 6). Medicine might well be one, but human society made it two.

Our understanding of the history of 'one medicine' as a movement remains patchy as does our knowledge of the entangled history of human and animal health. We have a promising sketch that suggests that the history of 'human' medicine was little more than a humanist fantasy. We find ourselves in a position to look again as we begin to see how animals were always present somewhere entangled in the web of modern medicine. But thus far our approach to the role of animals in health remains overly humanist, shackled to tired explanatory frameworks of institutions, professions, and society unthinkingly framed as all too human. Much more needs to be done if we are to understand what a more than human understanding of medicine and health may mean for our collective past, present and future.

ANIMAL AS MEDICAL OBJECT: RESEARCH AT THE BORDER OF HUMAN AND ANIMAL

Across the twentieth century, one of the most consistent – and contested – sites for the rapprochement of human and animal medicine was the scientific use of animals in biomedical research (Guerrini, 2003; Endersby, 2009). Twentieth-century medicine's close links to agricultural and particularly meat production was not restricted to public health concerns. On the contrary, slaughterhouses were a crucial resource for the early formation of 'biomedicine'. Amongst their lesser-known products were hormones and other 'biological' substances vital to early biomedical research (Pfeffer, 2010: 63–75). Here animals served as crucial resources for the experimental understanding of hormones and development of new endocrinological therapeutic innovations, not merely in death but also as 'tools' for the investigation and standardization of subsequent new therapies (Lederman and Burian, 1993; Clarke and Fujimura, 1992). Indeed, one of the comparatively understudied contributions of animals to modern medicine is in the early twentieth-century production, standardization and safety testing of the new biological therapeutics (Kirk, 2008). From the horse's role in the production of antitoxins, through the millions of rodents utilized for standardizing of therapies such as insulin, to the rabbits deployed for the safety testing of serum therapies to safeguard against serum sickness, modern scientific medicine is a multispecies enterprise. Nevertheless, historical attention has focused on the study of the role of animals in the production of medical knowledge rather than their place in the production of medical therapies (for a nuanced differentiation of the animal model from other experimental uses of animals, see Ankeny and Leonelli, 2011).

Early pioneers of bacteriology and immunology, including Emil von Behring, Paul Ehrlich, Robert Koch and Louis Pasteur, established the use of animals as models for the human as a paradigmatic tool in the scientific investigations of disease. Famously, Koch's principles made the creation of an animal model for a particular disease the 'experimentum crucis' for establishing a given factor as the cause of a given disease (Gradmann, 2017). Accordingly, as biomedicine cohered across the first half of the twentieth century, the routine use of animal models in scientific research 'linked human medicine inextricably with animals' (Bynum, 1990: 403). When Frederick Banting and John Macleod received the Nobel Prize in 1923 recognizing their identification of insulin, the role of dogs featured prominently in their respective Nobel lectures. Insulin provided the

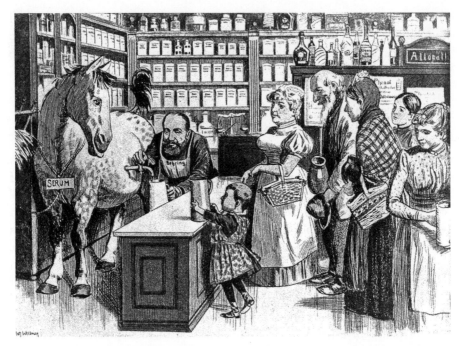

FIGURE 4.2: German Caricature showing von Behring extracting the serum with
a tap. Credit: Wellcome Collection.

first reliable treatment for diabetes and illustrates the way scientific medicine
entangled human health with the lives of animals. On the one hand, dogs were
central to the experimental work which linked insulin to diabetes (Bliss, 2007).
On the other, pharmaceutical companies manufactured insulin from animals
pancreases harvested from slaughterhouses. Furthermore, rabbits played a
crucial role in the manufacture of insulin, providing a means to standardize the
new 'biological' therapy to ensure accurate and safe doses could be administered
by physicians (von Schwerin et al., 2016). Across the twentieth century a variety
of species were drawn into the laboratory each perceived to be the best 'model'
for a particular research question. Fruit-flies were adopted as the quintessential
'standard' laboratory organism for early genetic research (Kohler, 1994), rats
were favoured by early behavioural scientists (Ramsden, 2011), mice were
established as the primary model for cancer research (Rader, 2004), dogs
provided a model for haemophilia (Pemberton, 2003) and the rhesus monkey
was employed by researchers working in infectious disease as well as
neurosciences (Blum, 1996; Hanson, 2004). However, the appropriation of
animals in the pursuit of human health was far from an unproblematic and
uncontested exercise. The biological boundary between human and animal was
not as porous as some within the biomedical sciences had hoped. Early

twentieth-century attempts to 'rejuvenate' human bodies through the transplantation of animal testicles proved as controversial as they were flawed (Hamilton, 1986). Attempts in the same period to graft animal skin to human bodies were equally contentious (Lederer, 2002). Even after immunology had developed as a specialism (Anderson and Mackay, 2014), what came to be known as 'xenotransplantation' continued to be pursued with the 1984 attempt to transplant a baboon heart into a human baby, a well-known and highly controversial example (Nathoo, 2009).

While it is notable that it was as problematic to establish cultural acceptance as it was biological in examples of the surgical transgression of the human-animal boundary, this is not to suggest that the successes of animal research met with societal approval. On the contrary, the experimental use of animals has been one of the most highly contested areas of modern medicine. In Britain particularly, the late nineteenth century had witnessed vociferous public debate about the social acceptance of animal research (Boddice, 2011; Rupke, 1987; Turner, 1980). The outcome was the passage of the Cruelty to Animals Act (1876), which established a British social contract for animal research that lasted for more than a century (French, 1975) but did little to silence its most vehement critics. Early twentieth-century resistance to animal research, or 'vivisection' as its objectors preferred to label the practice, focused on the dog – so much so that some leading scientific journals introduced more caution in the way research was reported if it involved experimentation on dogs (Lederer, 1992).

In Britain, the 1920s and 1930s witnessed a number of attempts to strengthen legislative protection for dogs or even exempt them entirely from scientific use. Similarly, across America, bills were presented in state legislatures while complex skirmishes occurred on the ground to determine access to stray animals. In response to such criticism, prominent scientists of the day were moved to defend the medical need for animals (Ross, 2015). Walter B. Cannon, for example, wrote a much-syndicated article titled 'The dog's gift to the relief of human suffering' (Cannon, 1926). The dog became the focus for antivivisection campaigns because it was perceived to be the most charismatic species most able to attract public sentiment. However, antivivisectionist discourse was also shaped by a number of concerns, not least those of class and gender (Finn, 2012; Lansbury, 1985; Kean, 1995). One prominent fear was that blurring biological boundaries between species would equally blur moral distinctions, leading to medical experimentation on humans (Lederer, 1997).

It is in the laboratory, in the experimental encounter, where scientific medicine is most clearly revealed as simultaneously working to undermine and sustain human difference to animals. For modern medicine gained scientific credibility from the evolutionary claim that animals exist on the same biological

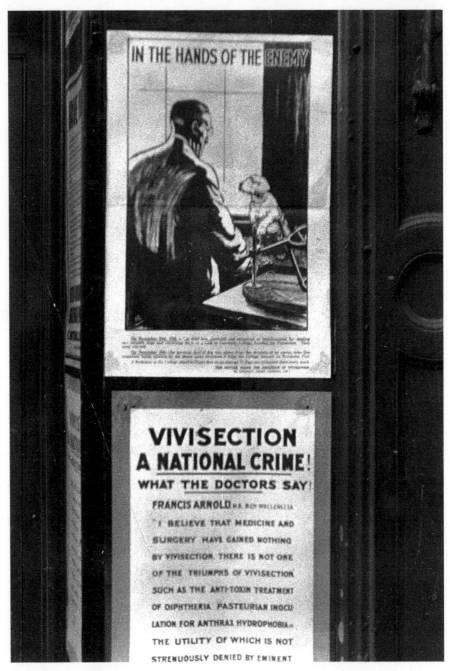

FIGURE 4.3: 'Vivisection: A National Crime', Anti-Vivisectionist Propaganda,
c. 1920. Credit: Wellcome Collection.

register as humans, while simultaneously claiming societal legitimacy from the moral claim that animals are to be located on a different ethical register to humans. The tensions inherent to the characterization of animals as biologically alike but ethically different to humans was arguably the most controversial aspect of modern medicine; however, it was also the most productive. Contesting and remaking the boundary between human and animal, within medical science and wider culture, drove not only the development of medical knowledge but also the making and remaking of understandings of human and animal difference and identity. Studying the history of humans, animals, health and medicine across the twentieth century reveals each to be interdependent upon and thus transformative of the other.

ANIMALS AS MODELS FOR THE HUMAN: THE CASE OF NONHUMAN PRIMATES

In 1945, the primatologist Robert Yerkes was invited to 'bring before one of the largest and most intelligent of radio audiences some indication . . . of the role which science can and should play in the new world'.[3] Titling his program 'Chimpanzees as servants of science', Yerkes explained that chimpanzees 'have high value as experimental animals' and were therefore 'bred and reared especially as servants of science to promote human welfare'.[4] The value of chimpanzees came from their biological and behavioural complexity which, Yerkes claimed, brought them so close to humans that they shared many physiological, cognitive and emotional characteristics. Evolutionary proximity to humans, therefore, made chimpanzees the ideal servant of science. Such thinking followed from the nineteenth-century work of Claude Bernard, whose principles continued to shape animal dependent biomedical science. Bernard had famously established:

> that to be really conclusive for man, experiments would have to be made on man or animals as near to him as possible . . . today, many people choose dogs for experiments, not only because it is easier to procure this animal, but also because they think that experiments performed on dogs can more properly be applied to man.
>
> —Bernard, 1957 [1865]: 122–3

One of the earliest examples of proximity to the human being mobilized to support the experimental validity of animal research on primates occurred at the Seventh International Medical Congress of 1881. Two conflicting experimental investigations of brain function were presented. Friedrich Leopold Goltz argued against cerebral localization (the belief that specific parts of the brain were linked to specific function), whereas David Ferrier claimed to have demonstrated the very same. Goltz presented evidence from his work on dogs from which the cortical substance of both the parietal and occipital lobes had been removed. The audience was invited to witness the animal's apparent normal behaviour and feel for themselves the large gaps in the animal's skull. In a similar way, Ferrier presented his research on monkeys that had undergone similar surgery. One monkey had lost all hearing while a second was unable to move the arms and displayed impaired movement of the legs. Ferrier drew on evolutionary proximity to explain the conflicting experimental evidence. '[T]he higher we go in the animal scale,' he argued, 'the greater the importance of the cerebral hemispheres.' Consequently, in dogs one witnessed 'comparatively slight and transient paralysis; whereas, in the monkey and man the paralysis is permanent' (MacCormac, 1881: 228–33). Goltz's mistake was to ignore the relative differences observed in 'higher' and 'lower' animals. Later, an expert committee killed and examined the animals, concluding that the damage to the monkey's brains was precisely what Ferrier had claimed whereas brain trauma in the dog was much less extensive that Goltz had believed. Brain localization was firmly established. So too was the conceptual presumption that nonhuman primates better represented the human. Subsequently, evolutionary theory was increasingly used to explain why primates should be the favoured animal for research into human neurological and behavioural pathologies more generally.

Societal factors also influenced the selection of nonhuman primates as favoured experimental models for humans. Animal dependent science, increasingly contested by a growing antivivisectionist movement, drew legitimacy from the claim that nonhuman animals accurately represented human pathologies (French, 1975; Rupke, 1990). Animal experimentation's acceptability was premised on its potential to produce positive therapeutic outcomes for human medicine. Accordingly, researchers should seek to work with species most likely to provide knowledge applicable to humans. On witnessing Ferrier's partially paralysed monkeys, for instance, Jean-Martin Charcot, the French neurologist, famously gasped, 'Mais c'est une malade' (It's a patient!) on recognizing in this monkey a gait that paralleled those he saw in human patients. Charcot's utterance was widely reported to underline the human need to experiment on animals. By enabling surgeons to locate and remove lesions from the brain, animal experimentation was cast as facilitating new treatments for human diseases. Ferrier's work was therefore frequently connected to human therapeutic benefits as a counter to antivivisectionist critique. In 1884, for instance, Ferrier's surgical techniques were said to have saved the life of a human patient whose continued existence was provocatively described as a 'living monument of the value of vivisection' (FRS, 1885). In this way, scientific practice and societal pressure combined to favour the use of nonhuman primates on the grounds that their evolutionary proximity to humans made them better models of human pathologies.

However, the scientific argument for the evolutionary proximity of nonhuman primates did not enhance their ethical status. On the contrary, in the late nineteenth-century popular imagination, ethical privilege was measured less in terms of evolution proximity to the human than in a presumed capacity to suffer. Propensity to suffer, in turn, was linked to the degree to which one was culturally civilized. Thus, the most civilized races were believed to have developed an increased sensibility to suffering, whereas the 'lower races' were thought to be less able to feel pain (Bending, 2000). Suffering was a property not so much of the biologically evolved but the culturally civilized. Consequently, social behaviour, alongside cognitive and emotional capacities, served as indicators for ethical inclusion. In Victorian Britain, this led dogs, above all other species, to be judged closest to humanity (having long been interwoven within human society and culture). As the physiologist and comparative psychologist George Romanes explained:

> The emotional life of the dog is highly developed – more highly indeed than any other animal. His gregarious instincts, united with his high intelligence and constant companionship with man, give to this animal a psychological basis for the construction of emotional character, having a more massive as well as more complex consistency than that which is presented even in the case of the monkey.
>
> —Romanes, 1888: 439

Dogs, therefore, were most capable of suffering and thus acquired privileged ethical status. Accordingly, the Cruelty to Animals Act (1876) asserted:

> an experiment calculated to give pain shall not be performed . . . on a dog . . . except . . . [when] the object of the experiment will be necessarily frustrated unless it is performed on an animal similar in constitution and habits to a . . . dog, and no other animal is available for such experiment.[5]

Horses, donkeys, asses and cats received the same privileged status: they could not be used if another species could serve in their stead. Ethical hierarchy was structured about shared social relations; each of these species featured prominently in day-to-day Victorian society. Consequently, popular opinion cared most for these species, ensuring they obtained privileged ethical status. Nonhuman primates were not privileged in this way until the late 1970s. The remainder of this article reconstructs how nonhuman primates became institutionalized with biomedical science and how, as a consequence, they became subjects of ever greater ethical concern.

Demand for purpose bred laboratory primates emerged in the first half of the twentieth century, responding to the gradual convergence of evolutionary and medical theory and the consequent material needs of biomedical research. New approaches to understanding and controlling infectious disease were critically important, such as the bacteriological work of Elie Metchnikoff (1845–1916), who pioneered an experimental evolutionary approach to infectious disease. Early bacteriologists found a number of major diseases, including syphilis, poliomyelitis and typhoid fever, could not be induced in conventional species of experimental animals. Metchnikoff explained these difficulties through evolutionary kinship. Whereas some diseases were widely shared across species, others were not. Accordingly, evolutionary proximity would increase the likelihood of a species sharing human disease. Metchnikoff demonstrated his theory by showing that chimpanzees were susceptible to a number of diseases that had hitherto proved impossible to replicate in nonhuman animals, including syphilis in 1903, baby cholera in 1908 and typhoid in 1910 (Krause, 1997). In Metchnikoff's work, experimental practice, conceptual understanding and evolutionary theory converged to make nonhuman primates, particularly chimpanzees, the favoured species for infectious disease research.

Nonetheless, working with nonhuman primates was challenging. In the early twentieth century, it was not possible to breed primates in captivity reliably, unlike most laboratory species (Yerkes, 1925). Instead, primates were caught in the wild and shipped from their native countries. This was an expensive and difficult process. Metchnikoff was uniquely situated to formalize an international supply network for primates as the Pasteur Institute (Paris) granted him substantial funding and eased access to French colonies in Africa. The Pasteur Institute's subsequent unparalleled access to chimpanzees, in large part due to having established a primate research and collecting station in Kindia, French Guinea, brought international recognition. For example, the Russian biologist, Ilya Ivanov, travelled to France and on to Africa in his early attempts to breed a human-ape hybrid (Rossiianov, 2002). Ivanov's experience led the Soviet government to establish the Sukhumi Primate Station in the southern Soviet Republic of Georgia, which became a leading centre for the production and use of laboratory primates (Fridman, 2002). Yerkes, in the United States, was similarly influenced, crediting Metchnikoff with inspiring his 'belief that the chimpanzee should prove uniquely valuable to biological investigators' (Yerkes, 1943: 292).

Metchnikoff, the Sukhumi Primate Station and the work of Yerkes are illustrative of the recognition that wild chimpanzees were far from ideal experimental animals. Purpose-bred chimpanzees produced in and for the laboratory were thought necessary if the scientific utility of chimpanzees was to be fully harnessed. As Yerkes explained, laboratory chimpanzees were to be shaped by their use:

> for problem solution. There is a very important, although often overlooked, difference between the study of an organism for itself and its use as a material

for problem solution. The former obviously emphasizes the importance of the organism; the latter, the importance of the problem which its use may help to solve.

—Yerkes, 1943: 291

Yerkes' 'laboratory colony' was very much intended to be just that: a colony of chimpanzees uniquely shaped for life in the laboratory. Historical studies have demonstrated the need to transition a species from a wild to a laboratory state so as to be useful within scientific research.[6] Excepting the phenomenal economic investment due to their size and lifespan, the chimpanzee was little different. Animals with valuable traits, not least docility, would have been chosen, bred and maintained for experimental use.

When Yerkes presented chimpanzees as servants of science, he did so in the knowledge that the argument for their utility to science might equally provoke moral questions about the legitimacy of such a role. He was aware of the ambivalent value of subservience. A servant is under obligation to work for the benefit of a superior and to obey their commands (servant deriving from the Latin *servus*, slave, which had particular resonance in the US). At the same time, entering into the service of another also carries positive value (for instance, when one enters into the service of the church or state). Yerkes wished to appropriate the idea of servitude in a similar fashion, so as to present the scientific use of chimpanzees in a positive light. Here, service is accompanied by the notion of sacrifice. Yerkes therefore spoke of chimpanzees being 'sacrificed to human need'.[7] When applied to the death of an animal within scientific discourse, 'sacrifice', then as now, evoked a positive and transformative meaning (e.g. Birke et al., 2007). However, voluntarily entering into servitude can be a noble sacrifice; to be forced into servitude is to enter a state of slavery. What sets apart positive from negative servitude is the ideal of free will. Accordingly, Yerkes was keen to emphasize how '[o]ne often feels the ape is enjoying his act', implying that laboratory chimpanzees engaged positively, quasi-voluntarily, with the obligations placed upon them by science (ibid., 2). By portraying chimpanzees in this way, Yerkes implicitly quelled moral objections to the scientific use of animals without directly engaging with such criticisms. If chimpanzees willingly collaborated with experimental procedures, who, then, could object to their role as servants of science?

Yet the constructed nature of laboratory primates invites us to question the meaning of acquiescence in this context. Whether human or nonhuman, Yerkes believed that behaviour was less the province of the individual and more the product of psychobiological factors that could be productively harnessed to shape the individual. He explained how 'studies of anthropoid apes and other experimental animals have gone far towards shattering the prevalent assumption or supposition that human nature cannot or should not be changed or improved' (ibid., 6). From this perspective, the question of willingly participation with experimental science is ambiguous. When Yerkes spoke of chimpanzees being 'bred and reared especially as servants of science', he had in mind practices that modified chimpanzees so as to render them servants of science. A guiding principle for producing laboratory primates was to render their behaviour compatible with experimental need (Hanson, 2004). Carl Hartman, for instance, who pioneered the development of laboratory Rhesus macaques in the 1920s, employed two 'chore boys' to 'handle' and thereby socialize his animals, to ensure that they accepted the experimental interventions encountered in the laboratory.[8] Indeed, Yerkes wrote the seminal guide to the production and management of 'standardized' laboratory chimpanzees (Yerkes, 1943). If chimpanzee behaviour could be modified to serve the needs of science more effectively, how, then, might a chimpanzee be said to 'acquiesce' to an experimental procedure? When laboratory chimpanzees are shown to be products of science, it is difficult to see how the principle of acquiescence can resolve the conflict between the scientific use of chimpanzees and growing ethical prohibitions against their use.[9]

Nevertheless, the importance of nonhuman primates to twentieth-century biomedical science and human health was soon established. In 1960, the National Institutes of Health established the Regional Primate Research Centers at the behest of the National Heart Institute, which had learnt that Russian scientists at the Sukhumi Primate Station had modelled hypertension in baboons. Despite being instigated by cardiology, nonhuman primates were framed as a necessary resource for all research:

> [T]o understand the nature of biological processes as they occur in man it is necessary to have available for research animals which resemble man as closely as possible. Many disease processes which occur in man can be studied only in man and subhuman primates. An outstanding example of this is poliomyelitis . . . this disease could not have been brought under control without an abundant supply of monkeys. Medical research is becoming more and more precise. Many research fields have gone almost as far as they can using lower animals, and progress lies in applying these methods and ideas to higher animals so that the relationship to man will be better understood.
>
> —Dukelow, 1995: 6

The use of rhesus macaques in the development of polio vaccine provided a powerful justification for investment in purpose-bred laboratory primates. There was every reason to believe that the increased use of purpose-bred laboratory primates would lead to further tangible benefits for human health. In the immediate decades following the close of the Second World War, such enthusiasm propelled the scientific use of nonhuman primates to its height.

Yerkes' public praise for primates as servants of science illustrates the absence of any substantial ethical concern for this species in 1945. The creation of purpose-bred laboratory primates, together with the scaling-up of laboratory primate use, contributed to enhancing the ethical significance of nonhuman primates in the decades after the Second World War. Maintaining large numbers of primates in captivity demanded rigorous knowledge of their welfare needs, in terms of physical health and, later, their social, cognitive and emotional well-being. Of critical importance in providing and systematizing knowledge of nonhuman primates was the new behavioural science of ethology (Burkhardt, 2005). Ethology placed strong emphasis on comprehending 'normal' animal behaviour as a precondition for experimental work. In 1959, for instance, the ethologist Robert A. Hinde questioned the possibility of making any sense of how an experimental intervention altered behaviour if one did not first understand normal behaviour (Hinde, 1959). By making knowledge of the normal behavioural repertoire of a species a condition of establishing a controlled experiment, ethology raised questions about the difference between purpose-bred laboratory animals and their 'natural' counterparts. Consequently, the use of laboratory primates in the latter half of the twentieth century was accompanied by substantial investment in field primatology, resulting in ever greater awareness of the psychological, biological and social complexity of nonhuman primate life. Hinde, for example, was funded by the British Medical Research Council to study the social behavioural needs of rhesus monkeys. In the mid-twentieth century, ethology was influential in shaping medical approaches to human behaviour and psychiatric well-being, not least through John Bowlby's 'attachment theory'.[10]

Hinde also supervised the PhD of Jane Goodall, whose ethological field studies of chimpanzees radically transformed scientific understandings of primate behaviour, as well as the place of nonhuman primates within the public imagination. Goodall was representative of a certain brand of ethologist who was keen to present their scientific work to a wide public audience. Goodall's *In the Shadow of Man* (1971), for instance, fundamentally changed chimpanzee's place in the public imagination by presenting the full complexity of their social life to a popular audience. Her work followed in the tradition of Konrad Lorenz (1952) and Desmond Morris (1968), whose cultural impact mirrored if not exceeded their scientific contributions. Goodall's compelling descriptions of chimpanzee society adopted an unashamedly anthropomorphic approach that would have been unusual to find in non-ethological scientific accounts of animal behaviour. Adopting a thoroughly humanizing narrative, such as the description of isolation suffered by a chimpanzee named Mr. McGregor as a consequence of having contracted polio, contributed to the transformation of the ethical status of chimpanzees. Working in the opposite direction, but with comparable effect, Desmond Morris's *The Naked Ape* (1968) applied ethological techniques to human society.

The work of ethologists such as Hinde, Goodall and Morris cannot be separated from the wider context of the increased use of primates within the experimental biomedical sciences. It was the experimental use of nonhuman primates which catalysed scientific interest in nonhuman primate life more generally. In 1962, for instance, Morris (1962) collaborated with experimental scientists in an attempt to establish the need for what he termed laboratory primate 'occupational therapy'. In this way, the nonhuman primates' role as a servant of science shaped a growing awareness of the complexity and importance of their cognitive abilities and social needs, which translated into greater concern for their welfare. One consequence can be found in the 1979 report of a UK governmental inquiry into the LD50 test, a particular contentious procedure subject to substantial criticism from the reinvigorated late twentieth-century animal advocacy movement. Quite outside its remit, and responding to the testimony of scientists and technicians who worked with laboratory primates, the report highlighted that:

> primates are in terms of evolution closer to man than cats or dogs and so possibly more likely to experience pain and apprehension to the same extent as a human being. Those who have worked with them, we are told, often feel a particular affinity with and sympathy for them which they do not feel for other species.
>
> —AACAA, 1979: 17–18

This led the UK government to extend the privileged ethical position that dogs, cats, asses and mules had possessed since 1876 to include nonhuman primates for the first time.

In the late nineteenth century, nonhuman primates, through presumed evolutionary proximity to humans, gained scientific but not ethical significance. Claude Bernard, for instance, having once vivisected a primate, refused to repeat the experience because he could not stand their physical resemblance to humans (Schiller, 1967). Yet his position was framed as a subjective dislike rather than an ethical stance. Over the course of the twentieth century, cultural understanding of the relationship towards, and understandings of, the presumed proximity of nonhuman primates to the human has changed. Nonhuman primates, perhaps more than any other nonhuman animal, possess significant ethical as well as scientific importance. Driving this change was an ever greater awareness of the degree to which anthropoid apes shared human-like social lives. Recognizing nonhuman primates as social beings formed a necessary condition for relating to these animals in ways that were more meaningful, morally and ethically, than had previously been possible. This process was driven in large part through the use of nonhuman primates as models for the human within the biomedical and behavioural sciences. Over time, humans, nonhuman primates, health, medicine and culture refashioned the other through complex, historically situated interdependencies. This is a process which Donna Haraway describes as 'situated histories, situated nature-cultures, in which all the actors become who they are *in the dance of relating*, not from scratch, not ex nihilo, but full of the patterns of their sometimes joined, sometimes separate heritages both before and lateral to *this* encounter' (Haraway, 2008: 25, emphasis original).

GENOMICS AND THE NEW KINSHIP

In the closing decades of the twentieth century, genomic science began to rewrite the book of life, making the genetic boundaries between species more porous than ever before (Kay, 2000). Genetic science, or genetic engineering, has primarily been developed and applied for medical ends. Genetically modifying mice, for instance, has allowed strains of mice to be engineered that model human diseases to a much higher degree of specificity. One of the first and most celebrated is 'OncoMouse', derived from a strain of mice genetically altered through the insertion of a gene that promotes cancer (an 'oncogene'). 'OncoMouse' is there predetermined to be highly susceptible to cancer providing biomedical science with a powerful new tool to study cancer and the factors that may cause or prevent the disease. OncoMouse is notable for a number of reasons. Created by a team of scientists at Harvard University with financial support provided by DuPont (an American-based global science company), OncoMouse was one of the first higher forms of life to be protected by patent (Jasanoff, 2005: 211–13). A transgenic organism, a hybrid of natural form and human culture, OncoMouse represents a new form of life created by biomedical science to serve as a biotechnological tool in the pursuit of health and profit. For Haraway, OncoMouse is also a 'Christ-like' figure for the new millennium, embodying the biomedical promise of humanity's secular salvation (Haraway, 1996: 46–7).

Genomic medicine embodies the entanglement of nature and culture, making their separation an evident fiction. Nowhere, perhaps, is this more evident than in 'Dolly' the sheep. Like OncoMouse, Dolly emerged from an academic-corporate partnership designed to harness the productive powers of animals for medical ends (García-Sancho, 2015). The aim was to transform agricultural animals by genetically engineering them to produce in their milk specific human proteins of biomedical value, which could subsequently be harvested and manufactured into therapeutic drugs. In order for such a process to be practically and economically viable, a means was required to mass-manufacture genetically transgenic animals from genetically engineered cells which were known to have taken up the desired human gene. Unfortunately, it was considered impossible to grow an animal from a cell. In the early 1990s, however, a group of scientists at the Roslin Institute, now part of the University of Edinburgh in Scotland, produced

Dolly as a demonstration that techniques for cloning animals could be developed and applied for this purpose (Wilmut et al., 2000). Dolly was not the first mammal to be cloned, though she was the first to be cloned from an adult cell. Hitherto, it had been widely believed that it was impossible to produce a clone from an adult cell. When presented to the public in 1997, the aim of harnessing farm animals for the production of human proteins for medical use barely registered. Instead, scientific, public and regulatory attention focused on the fact that Dolly had been cloned from an adult cell. The creation of Dolly challenged all manner of categories fundamental to humanism and the modern, including science and culture, human and animal, nature and artifice, medicine and agriculture, life and death. The world as it had been known would never be the same again.

Dolly changed not only what was possible within science but also the very fabric of cultural assumptions about mortality, reproduction and how families could be structured. Life after Dolly has been described by Sarah Franklin as a 'metamix of sex, in which the reproductive possibilities of plants, animals and microorganisms are conjoined with biotechnological expertise' (Franklin, 2007: 22). In the age of the clone, genealogy ceases to be linear, the facts of life become artefactual, parents multiply and new forms of kinship become possible – all, of course, at a price.

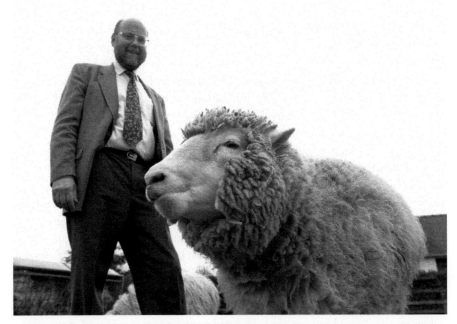

FIGURE 4.4: Scientist and Professor Ian Wilmut and Dolly, the world's first cloned sheep, at the Roslin Institute near Edinburgh where Dolly was developed and created. Credit: Colin McPherson / Contributor / Getty Images.

CONCLUSION: AN ECOLOGICAL VISION
OF HEALTH AND WELL-BEING?

In   *Modest_Witness@Second_Millennium.FemaleMan_Meets_OncoMouse:*
Feminism and Technoscience, Haraway (1997) identifies and deconstructs the
eponymous 'modest witness', which had served as the legitimate knowing
subject of modern science from the seventeenth century. The modest witness,
exemplified in Robert Boyle, established a specific subject (white, male), in a
situated position (impartial observer), within a particular space (the laboratory),
which allowed and legitimized the scientific production of objective knowledge.
Other subjects and forms of knowledge were excluded and thus disempowered.
At the dawn of the second millennium, as the twenty-first century approached,
this privileged modest witness had begun to unravel along with the figure of
man, as Foucault had earlier prophesied. Haraway described a possible
successor, FemaleMan, accompanied by OncoMouse, a 'sister mammal' which
is 'both us and not us; that is why we employ them' (Haraway, 1997: 82). With
FemaleMan and OncoMouse, Haraway creatively plays with new possibilities,
which embody and thus challenge the artificial dualisms animal and human,
nature and culture, male and female, us and not us. Such hybrids have always

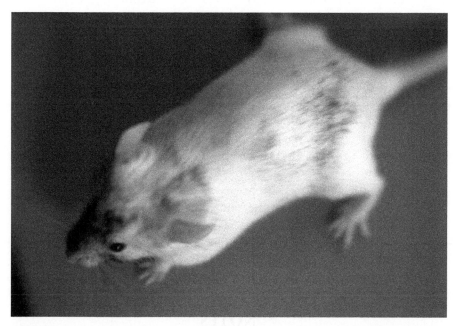

FIGURE 4.5: In this chimeric mouse the 2 component strains can be distinguished by
their coat colour. In this case the darker hair is derived from a parthenogenetically
activated embryo. Credit: Wellcome Collection.

been with us but only in passing from the modern to the postmodern have they become visible – even, as Thwaites becoming the GoatMan demonstrates, desirable.

The kinds of entanglement described in this chapter rest outside the conventional scope of humanist vision – perhaps even outside of modern history and found only in the postmodern. Nevertheless, to seek more than human histories of medicine is not to abandon the humanities as a way of knowing. On the contrary, it is to save them. Braidotti compellingly asks the humanities to recognize that humanism has imploded in the wake of the return of the nonhuman other. The consequent explosion of the anthropocentric premises which gave structure to the value system of humanism demands a response from the humanities which abandons nostalgia for what is lost in favour of opportunities to shape what can be won (2013: 143–50). For Braidotti, the 'proper subject' for the humanities is no longer 'man', but rather the possibilities embodied in the post-human (2013: 169 –73). This need not be the abandonment of the human but merely recognition of its historicity. Moreover, it is to frame a more humble human, respectful of and aware of its dependence on the other. Braidotti describes a 'new ecological posthumanism that . . . calls for self-reflexivity on the part of the subjects who occupy the former humanist center, but also those who dwell in one of the many scattered centers of power of advanced postmodernity' (2013: 49). Accordingly, a more than human history of medicine gestures towards the always tentative ecological interdependencies which make up the human and nonhuman animal. Across the twentieth century, health and well-being have been highly influential components in the making and remaking of human and animal. We might go as far as to begin to think about the twentieth century, of the modern, as having gifted the twenty-first century, the postmodern, an ecological vision of life, of health, of being and well-being together. Such a perspective invites the recasting of Lenin's question to respond to the postmodern: when we have never been human, what is to be done? (Haraway in Gane, 2006: 136). The future calls. What is the proper response of the historian? Rather than rallying against so-called anti-humanism, this chapter invites the cultural history of medicine to embrace the mere historicity of the human. In doing so, we can contribute to the remaking of medicine, the imagining of better ways of being human and the preservation of critical thought. As the humanistic arrangements of knowledge which hitherto sustained historical practice move inevitably into the past, we may still hope for a collective and better future.

NOTES

1. The notion that Osler coined the term 'one medicine' was apparently introduced in Saunders (2000). While Osler saw affinities between human and veterinary

medicine (particularly via comparative pathology), no evidence of his use of 'one medicine' has been traced. A recent attempt to clarify this question concluded that the most likely originator was Schwabe. See http://www.onehealthinitiative.com/publications/Who coined the term One Medicine by B Kaplan and C Scott May19 2011-CS.pdf . However, Bresalier et al. (2015: 8) have identified several earlier uses.

2. In Africa, partly as a consequence of human encroachment into what once was wilderness but now is an ever-dwindling landscape, traditional practices such as 'bush meat' consumption have been proposed as points for the introduction of HIV and Ebola into human populations (Sharp and Hahn, 2011).

3. 'Letter Warren Weaver to Robert Yerkes, 5/4/1945', Folder 1826, Box 96, Robert M. Yerkes Papers, Manuscripts and Archives, Yale University Library (hereafter RMY).

4. Robert M. Yerkes, 'Radio Broadcast Script, 4th May 1946', RMY.

5. 1876 An Act to Amend the Law relating to Cruelty to Animals Law Reports, Public General Statues, 39 & 40 Victoria c.77.

6. In particular, historians of science have emphasized the importance of 'standardization' animals so as to fit specific research cultures (e.g. Kohler, 1994; Rader, 2004).

7. Robert M. Yerkes, 'Radio Broadcast Script, 4th May 1946', RMY, p. 1.

8. I/159412 Hartman, Letter Carl G. Hartman to Meyer, 27 February 1935. Alan Mason Chesney Medical Archives, Johns Hopkins Medical Institutions, Baltimore, MD.

9. This is neither a historical nor a rhetorical point. In the early twenty-first century, the capacity of the animal to 'acquiesce' is increasingly proposed as an ethical condition for their participation in scientific research. See for example Altevogt et al. (2011: 3).

10. Bowlby, a British psychologist, psychiatrist and psychoanalyst, drew heavily from ethology and particularly the work of Konrad Lorenz in developing his ideas on the importance of maternal care (Vicedo, 2013).

CHAPTER FIVE

Objects

CORNELIUS BORCK

Modern medicine is full of objects. They come in many forms and sizes, from the simple first-aid kit with adhesive badges to the large technological system implemented for organ transplantation, including two operating theatres and the infrastructure delivering the organ from one to the other. A small pill suffices to intervene into human reproduction, and another is prescribed to regulate the behaviour of troublesome children. An X-ray reveals the interior of the body and tells the physician where to intervene into the body of a patient. Cochlear implants install hearing in deaf-born children and alienate them from the signing community of their parents. Modern medicine has always relied on tools and instruments, but over the last 100 to 150 years, medicine's objects have undergone an unprecedented evolution and multiplication. They have invaded society, driven the health industry, orchestrated large infrastructures and structured the political economy of health care. These objects intersect and interact with the body of the patient, rearrange social relations, embody medical knowledge, populate a doctor's office and guide medical treatment. In short, objects create and legitimate biomedicine. Today's medical practice focuses on the manipulation of bodies by instruments and the handling of technology for dealing with the human body. 'Medical technology makes up much of modern medicine' (Timmermann and Anderson, 2006: 1).

The history of modern medicine has often been told as the introduction of new tools and technologies,[1] starting with the invention of the stethoscope and the application of electrical currents in the nineteenth century or the clinical implementation of new diagnostic technologies such as X-rays and the ECG at the beginning of the twentieth century via ultrasound and CT scanning to the new imaging technologies towards the century's end. There is, however, no textbook on the history of medicine with a chapter on objects. Regardless of the dominance of tools and technologies in modern medicine, histories of medicine often took the construction of a diagnostic or therapeutic technology as an end in itself, to be evaluated within the context of medicine's objective aims and problems.

Twenty-five years ago, historian of medicine Harry Marks famously called on his colleagues to write proper life histories of medical technologies, including their often problematic dissemination and exploring the complex social implications that the implementation of an allegedly 'neutral' technology always entails (Marks, 1993). Meanwhile, science and technology studies, their related fields in history of medicine and medical ethnographies have started to work on medical technologies, placing their uses in the socio-cultural context (Lock et al., 2000; Stanton, 2002; Keating and Cambrosio, 2003; Burri and Dumit, 2007). Thereby, medicine's objects have found attention as powerful agents mediating life: they circulate widely in and out of the health sector; they get appropriated in unexpected ways as they interact with social and economic inequalities and political power hierarchies (Street, 2014; Gammeltoft, 2014; Sunder Rashan, 2017). Focusing on objects in a cultural history of modern medicine thus allows scholars to explore more generally the socio-political fabric the many and heterogeneous objects spin with their materiality along their construction, implementation and uses. In this chapter, I will combine insights from these studies with more conceptual and epistemological analyses of the way objects function in medicine as a scientific practice. The chapter also tracks how medicine's tools and instruments (themselves objects) interfered with medical knowledge and practice, driving a process of objectification of the human body that transgresses the realm of medicine.

THE STETHOSCOPE, AN OBJECT REPRESENTING MEDICINE

Technologically the stethoscope may appear to be a fairly inconspicuous tool, but it symbolizes professional medical expertise unlike any other object. In a recent 'A piece of my mind' contribution to the *Journal of the American Medical Association*, retiring cardiologist Lawrence Hergott described the packing-up of his stethoscope from the many objects in his office as the decisive moment for reflecting about his professional career:

It wasn't until about the fifth day, when I placed my 35-year-old stethoscope in a box, that tears came. Why then? I think tears came because, of all the artifacts I handled, the stethoscope was most symbolic of the connection I had made with the thousands of people to whom most of my adult life was dedicated. . . . Pondering my emotion over packing the stethoscope,

I realized that I was letting go of much more then what went into the boxes.

—Hergott, 2017: 137

Choosing the stethoscope for explaining his affection for the practice and the attachment to his patients, the retiring physician picked an object for communicating his humanistic appreciation of his profession. Although most of the stethoscope's diagnostic deliverables have meanwhile been delegated to more sophisticated medical technologies, this rhetorical gesture worked with remarkable ease, because this little instrument still functions as the paradigmatic signifier of professional medical practice. Along similar lines, medical students at the University of Lübeck can demonstrate their freshly acquired auscultation skills, in one of their public outreach activities, to the city's children in form of a teddy bear clinic offering an examination of the toy with the stethoscope. Likewise in many TV shows and screen productions, simply carrying casually a stethoscope around one's neck serves perfectly well for indicating a professional role in medicine. Reminiscent of the gesture of inspecting a glass of urine in early-modern paintings, the handling of a stethoscope functions today as the iconographic emblem of medical practice.

The stethoscope is a welcome starting point for analysing the multiple roles of objects in medical practice more generally and beyond its symbolic significance. Introduced by René Laënnec in the early nineteenth century, this object is obviously not an invention of the twentieth century, but its construction coincided with the beginning of modern medicine (Duffin, 1998). Already during the nineteenth century, the stethoscope altered its shape, morphing from a rigid wooden duct with two openings into a flexible tube with a soft membrane at one end and two earplugs at the other, but it still operates pretty much along the ways explained in Laënnec's early treatise (Laënnec, 1819). As a hearing aid, the simple tool introduced not only an instrument augmenting a human sense organ for diagnostic purposes, but also opened medicine to new ways of knowing, addressing directly the interior of the body (Sterne, 2003: 104ff). The classification of the diagnostic signs evoked in this process or their pathophysiological explanation may have changed, but the handling of the instrument and the transformation of medical practice it inaugurated has kept its significance – and points to the epistemological core of biomedicine. Looking at the practice of its use, the so-called auscultation, the stethoscope's mode of operation can hence be described as paradigmatic for modern medicine: the stethoscope connected body and ear by inserting a diagnostic interface between patient and physician in form of a material object. By doing so, the diagnostic tool changed the function of the oral communication between patient and physician and reorganized their interaction. The stethoscope started a direct interaction of the physician with the diseased body, where the physician had previously to rely on the observation of external signs and to talk with the patient about the experiences of an illness. For the new examination of the body, the instrument subordinated the patient to the commands of the physician performing the diagnostic process. The patient had now to keep quiet for not disturbing the examination and had to generate certain bodily actions like inspiration or expiration.[2] As a short formula for this new object-based form of medicine, it can be summarized that the patient had to shut up in order to let their body speak.

The invention of the stethoscope reorganized the interaction between patient and physician to a cultural *and* epistemological transformation of medicine, as the auscultation with the stethoscope became part of a new regime of physical examination. As a diagnostic tool, the stethoscope enabled further generations of objectification. Especially in the hospital, where the professional power hierarchies between physicians and their patients eased this mobilization of the body for examination and treatment, a new practice of medicine gained shape that continues to this day. In general, this was a shift away from the communication with the patient and towards the search for pathological signs by means of diagnostic instruments (Ackerknecht, 1967; Foucault, 1973).

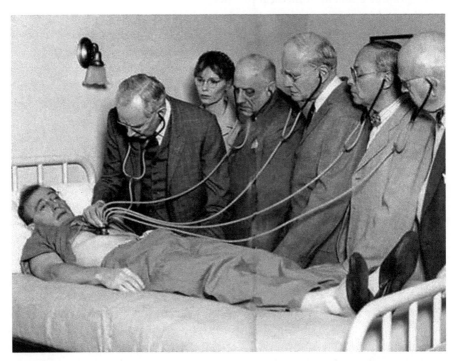

FIGURE 5.1: *Zelig*, 1983. Directed and written by Woody Allen, produced by Robert Greenhut and Orion Pictures, distributed by Warner Bros. Credit: Woody Allen, Robert Greenhut, Orion Pictures, Warner Bros.

According to Michel Foucault, *The Birth of the Clinic* started at the turn of the nineteenth century with a new epistemological regime, searching for the material substrates of diseases and linking clinical symptoms to pathological states as observed in the dead body by post-mortems that became a routine practice in the hospital during this period (1973). The new diagnostic process of the clinical examination bridged from the living, diseased body to the pathological states ultimately identified in the corpse as manifestations of a disease. The clinic as the new form of hospital medicine changed the social world of medical practice from a discourse on the individual experiences of an illness between patient and physician to the search for the objective substrates of particular diseases within the body. This was obviously a multifaceted process that affected the various sites of medical practice differently. The subjugation of the patients to the new regimes of clinical examination and bodily knowledge was most accentuated in the hospitals, which increased dramatically, in consequence, in number, size and institutional power. Comparing the current role of the hospital as the institutional and epistemic power centre of medicine with its older role since early modernity as a primarily social institution in urban life, the birth of the clinic captures an important cultural transformation, pushing more personal and holistic forms of healing to the margins.

The invention and introduction of the stethoscope did obviously not steer this transformation on its own, but participated at this process in many ways, serving as a medium along the multiple meanings of this term:[3] most immediately, the stethoscope mediated between the body of the patient and the physician's ear, transmitting otherwise inaudible sounds from the body's interior to the listening physician. In this process, the subjective signs of suffering became linked to objective symptoms of diseases, thereby opening medicine to a new epistemic space and reforming medical knowledge. At the same time, the instrument rearranged the patient-physician relationship, choreographing their interaction and replacing oral communication with silent obedience for detecting objective signs of clinical conditions as bodily diseases. In addition, the instrument required new examination skills, rearranging professional training towards the handling of instruments that increasingly determined objectified disease entities. The stethoscope started medicine's objectifying gaze. Over time, it symbolized the prestige of the new professional expertise in handling objectified diseases, distributing power along the hierarchical layers of the health system. The stethoscope, one of modern medicine's more simpler tools, thus testifies to the complex interweaving of theory and practice, social relations and biomedical alterations, institutional power and individual experience. The stethoscope can be described as a piece of technology that guided a transformation of medical practice towards objectified knowledge.

When objectification can be ascertained as the fundamental mode of operation of current medicine, how has this mode changed in relation to the history of objectivity? In their seminal study comparing scientific atlases from the eighteenth century onwards, Lorraine Daston and Peter Galison differentiated three different styles of scientific accuracy relating to three distinct ideals of empirical knowledge and scientific ethos (2007): whereas atlas makers around 1800 printed idealized objects for depicting them true to their essential 'nature', the scientific community shifted during the middle of the nineteenth century towards 'objective' images, in which even the most incidental details had not been deleted, in order to demonstrate a strict abstinence from any subjective manipulation. Still later, the images started to highlight particular patterns in the name of a 'trained judgement', guiding the observers' attention. Since Daston and Galison included in their study medical atlases, this chapter can follow their general argument and trace how objectivity was implemented in medical research as epistemic virtue in the course of the nineteenth century.

Looking more specifically at the role of objects in medical practice, however, an important difference to the history of objectivity as reconstructed by Daston and Galison becomes apparent: in contrast to science in general, and its *Images of Objectivity* in particular, medical research is tied to the treatment of individual patients. It has to address the scientific as well as socio-cultural complexities of real-life problems in individual patients, and hence faces particular problems in the translation between laboratory models, basic scientific research and clinical situations. Partly in response to these problems, partly because of economic pressures to increase efficiency, a new ideal of empirical knowledge has been implemented in clinical practice as epistemological framework towards the end of the 20th century (Cochrane, 1972; Berg and Timmermans, 2003). With the introduction of evidence-based medicine (EBM), the experts' trained judgement no longer suffices as legitimization for a therapeutic intervention and has been replaced by efficiency studies on therapeutic interventions and by clinical guidelines, synthesizing the available empirical evidence from large clinical trials and other forms of statistical surveys to recommendations for clinical decisions (Gifford, 2011; Borck, 2016; see also Greene's chapter, 'Disease', in this volume). The new ideal of empirical knowledge takes objectification to the level of the collective for addressing the individual patient. With EBM, medicine's objectifying gaze that started with the stethoscope has meanwhile arrived on a plane where all forms of biomarkers are fed into statistical analyses together with measurements of the quality of life or of individual experiences. Medicine's ultimate object is now the datum (cf. 'The virtualization of medicine and its re-appropriation' later in this chapter).

MACHINES AS MEDICINE'S PROSTHESES

Medicine's mobilization of technology did not go unnoticed and unchallenged. Already during the early decades of the twentieth century, physicians and other voices critiqued it as a mechanistic and reductionist form of machine medicine, subjugating patients to the technical routines of the machines employed (Lawrence et al., 1998). The factory-like operation of the modern hospital epitomizes an alienation of the patients from their personal lives, this line of critique seems to imply treating them as anonymous units just like the hospital gown highlights their de-individualization. For fully embracing such a general conclusion, however, a cultural history of medicine should evaluate the epistemic efficiency of this objectification at work in medicine. Investigating more closely how patients are turned into objects of medical procedures reveals the functioning of the machine model as the operative core of medical practice and its centre of efficiency. Davis Baird has argued that scientific things are much more than mere material objects as they encapsulate knowledge. The instruments and machines of scientific research have to be understood as materialized forms of knowledge (Baird, 2004). Building on his analysis, this section describes how medical practice relies on such knowledge machines: they are constructed and implemented for constituting powerful representations of the body.

The many machines, tools, tests and instrumental procedures mobilized for and utilized in medical practice point to its operative core in material and epistemological terms. In today's technologized medicine, objects are not mere things used in its practice; medicine has become objectified in a much more fundamental sense: diagnostic instruments register data of all sorts for generating objective representations of diseases which are then targeted by therapeutic interventions with more instruments. In the new visual cultures of medicine, the three-dimensional body is, for example, often rendered on the two-dimensional plane of the photograph or computer screen, requiring new visual conventions for connecting medicine to the images of objectivity as described by Daston and Galison. Along such lines, Barry Saunders has described the complex technical as well as epistemic and social work going into the implementation of CT scanning for arriving at diagnostic evidence (2008), the technical components have to be adjusted to the details to be depicted by the new technology and these have to be aligned with the knowledge about diseases, and the medical practice needs to be adapted, in order to make the representations generated by the CT machine (itself a materialized form of knowledge) translate between the individual body, the diagnosis and a therapeutic intervention.

Although visualizations play a dominant role in current medical practice, other diagnostic technologies translate states of diseases to mere numbers, from simple measurements of height and weight to sophisticated blood analyses. Along these different ways, diagnostic machines generate objective representations of diseases, which then guide and legitimize possible therapeutic interventions. The representations mediate between a patient's experience of an illness and their body, between the individual body and medical knowledge, between the knowledge and the therapeutic intervention, between the actions of the physician and the health insurance, between the patient and the hospital administration, between the client and their employer, etc. Medical practice does not only rely on tools and technology, but revolves around the disease representations derived with these means from the body. Representations have become the central objects of medical practice today.

An extreme, but paradigmatic case for elaborating on this case is minimally invasive surgery where the operating instruments are inserted together with a visualization device into the body: while the cutting knife or the suturing needle moves through the flesh, the centre of control has moved during the operation from the open and exposed body to the representational spaces on the screens monitoring the procedure. Here the representations have literally become the targets of medical practice. The implementation of these new technologies obviously relies on a massive re-learning that includes the entire personal working in medicine, but also the patients who are confronted with these technologies and who now have to translate between their technologically mediated experiences and their needs, beliefs and wishes (Prentice, 2012). Pinhole surgery thus provides the paradigmatic case of current medical practice, where the handling of instruments and the manipulation of objects on screens have moved to the centre.

This form of objectified medicine functions best where the matching between patient, body and representations can be tightly controlled, e.g. in the operating theatre or the intensive care unit. In these particular spaces, the thing knowledge of medicine has arrived at another level, as representation does not stop here with visualization and monitoring, but also works literally by re-presentation, with machines taking on the roles of bodily organs. Machine replicas of bodily organs in form of artificial respiration, blood filtration or perfusion step in for physiological functions, sometimes for brief moments, sometimes for the rest of the life. The machines re-presenting bodily organs complement medical practice as prosthetic hybridizations. The construction of prostheses as artificial replacements of human organs or bodily functions can be described, in this epistemological perspective, as a paradigmatic example of the efficacy of modern medicine. Relying on the objectifying gaze of the representational practices, the prosthetic hybridization of therapeutic interventions characterizes medicine as a machine practice.

With the implementation of machine replicas in clinical practice, a popular vision of the human body as a machine seems to have become reality. Already in the 1920s, Fritz Kahn depicted the human body in such a way as an 'industrial palace' with all sorts of machines replacing bodily organs: the heart is a pump, the kidneys a filtration system, the lungs a ventilation apparatus, etc. Thanks to the myriad developments in engineering and biotechnology, medicine's machinery may no longer resemble the industrial age, but the programme is still

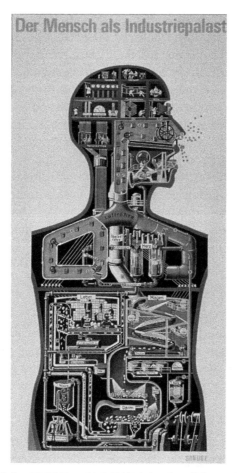

FIGURE 5.2: Fritz Kahn, Der Mensch als Industriepalast (Man as Industrial Palace), 1926. Credit: © Kosmos Verlag.

valid. It is a programme that guided the development of the biosciences since the 'experimentalization of life' in the nineteenth century (Rheinberger and Hagner, 1993). The 'human motor' had formed the conceptual basis of experimental physiology, catalyzing its rise to the status of a leading research programme and contributing to the rise of modernity's regimes of production (Rabinbach, 1990). With the arrival of the first prosthetic hybridizations such as the 'iron lung' or the artificial kidney, the conceptualization of the body as machine turned into a new therapeutic opportunity and reinforced the reductionist understanding of the human body as a technological system. Since then, the human body may no longer resemble an industrial palace, but machine medicine has advanced to become a major business sector and has certainly become an industry.

Kahn's popular image of the human machine as an industrial palace also sheds some light on the divergent social alliances of the concept (Kahn, 1931). The body as machine and the hospital as factory may amount to a common dystopia for many critics, but Kahn and others envisioned it as the basis for a new technological humanism. For Kahn, medicine's objectification of the human body to a machine explicitly served his liberal agenda of enlightening the society about human nature: Because perfect machines can in principle replace all bodily organs, the human body no longer remains a mysterious object but can be appropriated (Borck, 2007; Sappol, 2017). Visualization followed here the strategy to combine the popularization of medical knowledge with a firmly established belief about the promise of technology for medicine. The image conveyed expectations not only of a technologically perfected medicine but also of a thorough understanding of human nature, because machines were completely explainable. The British biologist J. Z. Young followed the similar strategy, when he explained in his *Doubt and Certainty in Science*:

> Comparison of living things with machines may seem at first to be a crude, even rather childish procedure, and it certainly has limitations; but it has proved to be extraordinarily useful. Machines are the products of our brains and hands. We therefore understand them thoroughly and can speak conveniently about other things by comparing them with machines.
>
> —Young, 1968: 22

In addition to 'understanding [the body] thoroughly' and speaking 'conveniently about [it] by comparing [it] with machines', as described by Young for biological research, machine organs can be employed in medicine as prosthetic hybridizations, as described above. However, the powerful dynamics in the cultural exchanges between bodies and machines do not stop there. If a bodily organ can be perfectly well conceived as a technological object, it can be optimized and perfected like any other thing. In addition to the long-lasting debate on the question whether machine medicine implies an inhumane mistaking of a living being for a technological system (Lee, 2012), the objectification of the human as a machine rests on a culturally problematic epistemology that unleashes the idea of optimization (Borck, 2012): as a machine, the human becomes an apparatus open to optimization. With prosthetic hybridization, the perfect machine becomes the ideal for the human body and the human is turned into a project of constructive optimization (Harasser, 2016). The concept of the cyborg derived from the astronautics of the 1960s and 1970s, the prime time of the technological fix for every possible problem, but the cyborg did not stay within the realm space research (Barfield, 2015). Like the human machine, it became a popular figure pointing to the dimension of enhancement intrinsic to modern medicine. With prosthetic hybridization, enhancement in the form of the technological or pharmacological optimization of the human body can no longer be described as something alien and conceptually totally different to therapeutic medicine (Eilers et al., 2014). Enhancement is the path opened by machine medicine's prostheses.

According to the promise of technologized medicine, representations capture everything of the patient that is needed for the procedure. The representations on diagnostic screens, monitors or in the patient record objectify the disease to a manageable thing, legitimize the therapeutic actions and guide their realization. Even in cases where something goes wrong, this happens on the representational level, where a monitor visualizes a failed procedure, a light starts to flash or an alarm sounds. How closely and tightly prosthetic hybridization captures medicine's mode of operation can be clarified further by looking at cases where this approach fails. Obviously not all forms of medical treatment rely on objectifying representations and prosthetic hybridization. Training, rehabilitation, dietary regimes or simply rest still form an important part in healing processes, but it is no coincidence that these approaches have lost their prominence in contemporary medicine. In situations and contexts where prosthetic hybridizations are not available, because the representational grip is less tight or fails to capture the specificities of a situation of suffering, modern medicine simply does not function well.

Take the example of pain, a very common complaint and many often the reason for seeking medical help. There have never been more effective remedies for pain from analgesics to anaesthesia than today, but chronic pain has nonetheless turned into a major health issue in all Western societies and is the main reason for early retirement. Pain is a subjective experience and there is no objective biomarker for it. The experience of pain can easily be measured by rating scales, but all attempts to link these scores to biological alterations as determined in the representational spaces of biomedicine have failed. In addition, the easy access to effective pain-relief pharmaceuticals also appears to worsen the long-term consequences of the condition.

The example can be gradually generalized to other conditions of suffering where the representations of a patient in terms of objectified disease states do not match well with the patient's situation, as in chronic or ill-defined ailments. In these instances, where the representational mode reaches its limits, modern medicine encounters enormous difficulties or fails. In the interstices between human illness and suffering on the one hand and medicine's operation by prosthetic hybridization on the other, various forms of appropriation, of tinkering with medicine's always only partial solutions, take place, because the perspective of the objectified machine entails severe limitations when addressing the suffering body of the ill patient (Mol, 2008). Paradoxically, such tinkering with medical objects to adapt them to individual needs also applies to prostheses, e.g. the cases where medicine's mode of prosthetic hybridization offers an artificial replacement. Regardless of the new prominence of high-tech artificial limbs in popular culture and advertising as perfect and stylish tools, the users of these appliances typically appropriate the technological thing by tinkering, with the eventual aim of being able to forget about them (Sobchack, 2006).

SEEING IS BELIEVING

The name 'stethoscope' was, strictly speaking, a misnomer. Laënnec labelled it a tool providing visual access to the interior of the chest, although the instrument functioned acoustically. The strange name 'stethoscope' highlights yet another aspect of modern medicine's object culture – its reliance on visualization. In a way, the name was a fortunate mistake, as the new diagnostic tool started medicine's participation at the 'scopic regimes of modernity' (Jay, 1988). Since the last century, modern medicine has become a highly visual affair, even though most of its targets are concealed in the body's interior or of a size far too small for inspection by the natural eye. The objectifying regimes of representational medicine produced ever more kinds of visualization, magnifying the objects searched for, depicting new entities by penetrating the body with rays, waves, tracers or instruments – or by visualizing constructs invisible by nature such as time courses of electrical currents. Take, for example, the record of the heart's electrical activity, the electrocardiogram (ECG): the pattern of an initial slow and small wave, followed by a large, brief, bipolar peak and a larger, longer wave, the PQRS-complex, is well established as the physiognomic image of a healthy heartbeat, and yet it exists only as a techno-scientific construct of a by nature invisible entity that required enormous work not only in engineering but also for the standardization of the technological procedure, for connecting the recorded traces with disease categories and adapting the existing understanding of heart diseases, and also for translating the patterns in the communication with the patients. The image of the healthy heartbeat demonstrates by its characteristic pattern how visualization depends on the conventions implemented for recording it in internationally standardized ways – historically a long and cumbersome process (Howell, 1996).

With regard to the current dominance of visualization in medicine, it is important to notice how visualization regimes not only render visible objects concealed in the body's interior but also generate images of objects invisible by nature in material as well as epistemic terms. Many objects of modern biomedicine rely in this way on sophisticated visualization strategies. The technological ensemble of the recording instruments and the algorithms for data selection, filtering, analysis and display construct visible entities that are at the same time the real product of the machines and of the work stabilizing the objects generated by the technology. Modern biomedicine thus testifies to the character of the modern (techno-) sciences to operate as 'phenomenotechniques', as Gaston Bachelard described them (Bachelard, 1934; Rheinberger, 2005): they construct 'surreal' entities according to their technical rationality (Kotowicz, 2016). Because of the constructive efforts necessary for constituting these visual entities, visualization in medicine cannot be understood as a form of re-presentation of something existing 'out there' in nature, even if it is depicted on a photograph. Only the visualization process itself brings the depicted entity into existence; the technologies mobilized for its production mediate between material constraints and social conventions and format its epistemic specificities.

Modern visualization procedures hence go far beyond picturing what is out there by shaping and forming the depicted object. This is important to highlight in order to understand the constructive potential of visualization as a crucial part in the cultural context of research and practice. The visualization of an object takes always a specific perspective, it has to select a suitable target, and its complex nature is further effectuated by power relations, economic accessibility and social demand. Objectification by visualization coevolves with technology but does not stop at the limits of the human senses nor at the borders of the physical world. It unfolds along the possible worlds of the artifactual construction of images as representations of diseases. It stops at the limits of engineering and human imagination or with the legibility of the visualizations generated. This has made visualization such a powerful tool for research, especially in the life sciences. Visualization has hence become a massively studied topic in science and technology studies, exploring how the rationality of scientific visualization is embedded in complex social contexts and enacted in specific, often locally contingent cultures and practices (Lynch and Woolgar, 1992; Coopmans et al., 2014; Carusi et al., 2015). In addition, many visualization techniques are costly procedures, linked to powerful interventions into the body and society (Cartwright, 1995; Kevles, 1997). These local and cultural contexts of mediation anchor visualization also in the human lifeworld with its fabric of anthropological and philosophical conceptualizations (Dijck, 2005; Borck, 2018; Vall, 2009), as the biological specifications of the targeted object may differ enormously from a patient's experience of suffering from an illness.

A telling example of how biomedical visualizations intervene as objectifying images into the complex social fabric of a patient's personal life is given by Simon Cohn, listening to a psychiatric patient describing the relevance of an fMRI scan of his brain:

> The scan is important because it shows just what has been wrong with me all these years . . . you don't have to listen to descriptions or anything, you can see it there before your very eyes. [. . .] I have bipolar, and I have done for

years. It's who I am, and I can't imagine not suffering from it. So, you see, I don't want to suddenly wake up and not be a bipolar . . . What I want is to be able to say to people, ‚Look. This bit of my brain, that's why I am bipolar. But I am bipolar, so if I have to live with it, why can't you?'

—Cohn, 2012: 188

The patient may not have 'read' the scan in a medically appropriate way, but the images made sense to him in a much more straightforward way. The patient immediately understood the mode of operation of visualization in biomedical research, e.g. yielding hitherto inaccessible objects full of significance for research and medical practice as well as for the individual life of the patient. Here, the objectifying gaze of technoscientific medicine turned highly subjective suffering into something objective and instrumental for further social interaction.

This holds also true for the circulation of such images among psychiatrists and neuroscientists: images provide evidence required for research publications, further studies and public discourse. Thereby the visualizations shape the understanding of psychiatric conditions along the path of the technically generated representations of disease states that have been developed along the socio-political path of engineering, they guide therapeutic interventions into problems identified as effective targets for treatment and form a technologically mediated conceptualization of psychiatric suffering. In *Picturing Personhood*, Joe Dumit has elaborated on the various assumptions that went into the constructions of such brain scans and on the many negotiations required for constituting the entities made visible by the new technology as appropriate objects of psychiatric research and treatment (2004). Brain scans also demonstrate how biomedical visualizations work outside of medicine, as Cohen's patient and Dumit's book make clear: they circulate widely through society and popular culture, they intervene in patients' lives or they can serve as evidence in courtrooms.

The brain scan objectifying 'being bi-polar' and offering its appropriation to a patient points to both the ready acceptance of such visualizations by the allegedly lay people and the wide circulation of biomedical representations in the public sphere. In this twisted way, the episode provides a striking example for the process once described as medicalization, the transformation of human experiences and problems into medically defined conditions (Illich, 1975). Yet the example demonstrates how the concept captures only partially what is going on, as the process does not stop with labelling a psychic disturbance a disease. The patient was not the mere victim of an all-powerful medical industry but re-appropriated the medically objectified condition in unanticipated ways. The classic concept of medicalization with its clear dichotomy between power and dependency has to be complemented by ethnographic, socio-political and material analyses of how such power asymmetries get established and can be negotiated, maintained or transformed. Biomedical visualizations are powerful images; their political, institutional, social and epistemic effects cannot be deduced from the entities objectified in the image or from medicine's dominant position in the health system or the evidence for the efficacy of a therapeutic intervention. Biomedicine's objects offer their utility to the various actors in the health sector in many heterogeneous ways, and 'biomedicalization' has to be studied as a complex process involving the society at large (Clarke et al., 2010).

The complex social implications of diagnostic technologies are particularly problematic in the field of prenatal testing where a termination of the pregnancy instead of effective treatment is the consequence. Rayna Rapp has presented a very careful and compelling account of the complex interactions entailed by the seemingly objective diagnosis of an unborn foetus with Down's syndrome (2000). Including in her study not only patients from various classes, religions and ethnicities but also counsellors, gynaecologists, obstetricians and technicians, Rapp details the social work going into the fabrication of the diagnosis in the laboratory and disentangles the many communication failures between counsellor and patient, in addition to describing the massive social impact of the diagnosis. Many problems for the counselling obviously derive from differences in language and scientific literacy, but more profoundly, they arise from differences in philosophy and culture. Medicine's ethical imperative of the informed consent remains its ultimate goal but can never be fully accomplished, as she convincingly shows. Patient belief systems are too complex to be understood completely within the setting, especially in the case of prenatal testing where beliefs of family values, concepts of parenthood, beliefs about the status of the foetus, the meaning of risks and the nature of disability are at stake.

The medicalization of pregnancy has a long history, making it an apt topic for studying the transformative powers of the objectifying gaze of medical technologies. Contrasting the current regimes of surveillance, testing and monitoring with a careful analysis of the notes by a physician from the eighteenth century, Barbara Duden has traced how the medicalization of pregnancy turned a natural phase of human female life into a problematic and dangerous period requiring constant medical attention, and how this process affected both the individual experience and the socio-cultural valence of pregnancy (1991). In addition, the medicalization of pregnancy interfered with well-established gender roles, changing the culture of childbirth, repositioning the social space of midwifery and turning large parts of its domain into (initially exclusively male) obstetrics. Exposing the long-standing and continuing gender bias of medicine, the medicalization of pregnancy became an obvious target for critique from the women's health movement (Nelson, 2015).

There can be no doubt that the new regimes of prenatal monitoring and of reproductive medicine massively affected and altered the biological conceptualization, psychic experience, social organization, material practice and cultural understanding of pregnancy and human reproduction during the twentieth century (Pfeffer, 1993). The image of a syringe injecting sperm into an egg cell has turned into an iconic representation for the powers of reproductive medicine – meanwhile a massive and global industry. The omnipresence of this image, which does not show very much as it zooms in on the details of a lab procedure, nonetheless illustrates an important aspect of the dynamics of objectification in

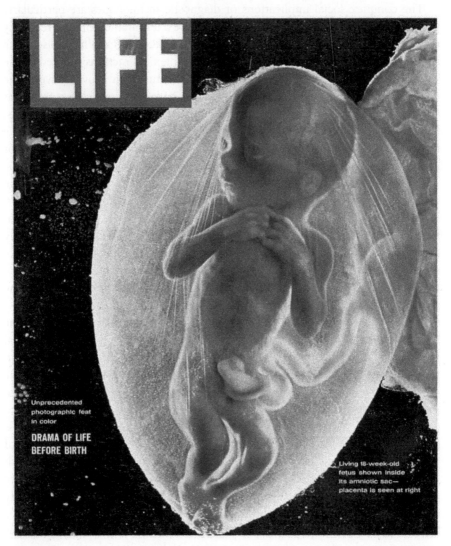

FIGURE 5.3: First picture of a human foetus published in the press (Cover of *Life*, 1965, picture by Lennart Nilsson). Credit: Editorial Image Provider / Contributor / Getty Images.

biomedicine: many of its targets, especially in the domain of genetic testing and reproductive medicine, escape the limits of visibility. At the core of the scopic regimes of modern medicine rests the domain of the invisibly real, though not in the sense of a Freudian concept or transcendental essence, but in the very material form of surreal medical objects – like the gene for an inherited disease of which not even the geneticist can determine whether it will affect the unborn child.

It is instructive to compare these more recent images from reproductive medicine with the first photographs of unborn human life that hit the public in the mid-1960s. Lennart Nilsson's famous images showed an isolated unborn human shining in a fleshy and warm rosy against a dark sky at night with some stars, thereby signifying the promise of a future life. And yet he had arranged aborted foetuses by sophisticated background illumination to eye-catching portrayals of the wonders of life in a sentimental narrative of the scientific discovery (Nilsson, 1966; Jülich, 2015). Nilsson's photographs demonstrate in a very drastic way how radical the conveyed meaning can differ from the depicted object. His images thus testify inadvertently to the powers of the iconographic traditions and visual conventions he carefully employed (with a bright and warm colour indicating the value of life, for example). In addition, his images separated the foetus from its environment in the pregnant body, from its unity with the mother, thereby paving the way for the political debate on the status of the embryo as autonomous subject. His spectacular images made global headlines, and in 2015 the TIME magazine included it in its list of the 'most influential images of all time'.[4] Nilsson's photographs thus testify to the power of medical representations in today's culture. His images of hitherto invisible objects (the baby to come) were attributed with notions of autonomy and person-like individuality that had traditionally been restricted to living people, and that certainly contradicted with the destructive process of the taking of these photographs. Nilsson's images acted as 'immutable mobiles' described by Bruno Latour (1986): they forged new and unlikely alliances by their transportation into different socio-political contexts. Anti-abortionists, for example, took up Nilsson's images as visual tools for celebrating life in aggressive 'pro-life' campaigns (Petchesky, 1987; Morgan and Michaels, 1999). The objectifying gaze that started with the stethoscope and resulted in biomedicine's visual cultures engaged science and society with the powers of visualization. The images took on many different roles both within and outside of medicine.

HEALTH MATTERS: EXHIBITING MEDICINE BY ITS OBJECTS

Medicine's numerous objects and its immersion in a visual culture offered themselves for display and for alliances within an emerging market of health exhibitions. Anatomical collections enjoy a long history as places of display and study, and during the nineteenth century they were complemented by anthropological museums, aligning them with the biopolitical agenda of racial hygiene (Knoeff et al., 2015). The opening of the First International Exhibition on Hygiene in Dresden in 1911, however, signalled a new era of educational practice in public health, focusing on the display of medical objects. Combining innovative visualizations of human anatomy and physiology with information about health prevention, the Dresden exhibition attracted visitors in large numbers and set the tone for a new form of health propaganda, kindling exhibitions with similar ambitions in many countries (Nikolow, 2016). Together with pamphlets, posters and films, the health exhibition quickly became a major new medium of medical education in the twentieth century, addressing school classes, soldiers and workers, and also the general public. Putting medicine on display by exhibiting its objects became a massive undertaking for educating the public about basic guidelines for a healthy life in a patronizing form of biopolitics.

In their efforts to exhibit the advances of modern medicine and to educate the public about the basic principles of health prevention, medical exhibitions became an important arena for public health and health education. Particularly in this space of collective attention, modern medicine collectivized bodily

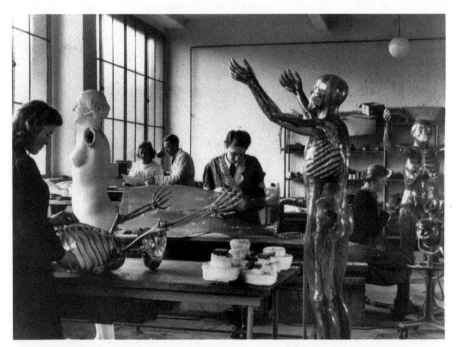

FIGURE 5.4: Production of the Famous Men of Glass, Dresden Hygiene Museum, *c.* 1950. Credit: Deutsches Hygiene-Museum.

health to a common good, moral value to society and hence as a common concern on the collective level (Usborne, 1992). Masses attended these shows – the hygiene exhibition in Dresden had attracted 5 million visitors – and the masses became the declared target of medicine, most significantly by complementing individual health with the well-being of the collective body of the (racialized) nation. A most powerful driving force for this discourse was the theory of evolution and its translation into eugenics. Propagating the betterment of the human race, eugenics quickly turned to the negative in the twentieth century in the context of fears of degeneration and fierce national rivalries (Kevles, 1985; Paul, 1995).

Eugenics culminated in the Nazi holocaust and euthanasia programme for mentally ill patients (Weindling, 1989). The *Volkskörper*, the national body conceived as the biological entity defining the nation's future health, subverted medicine's care for patients by an attention to the collective body as medicine's perverted final aim. Under the shadow of the catastrophe the Nazi regime had brought, Edward Steichen curated the *Family of Man* exhibition at the MoMA in New York in 1955 as an antidote to racial hygiene, focusing on the commonalities of people from all cultures. Originating from the intention to counter racism, the exhibition again addressed the collective body of mankind and used photography as the allegedly universal language for propagating this message: the collective body was, perhaps, modern medicine's and modernity's most uncanny object.

A telling example of the difficulties medical museums faced with the miniaturization of biomedical objects is the Wellcome collection in London. It started in the twentieth century with collections of medical objects and instruments from previous times and foreign cultures, for illustrating how medicine had changed to the better (Engineer, 2000). The central role of objects in its practice opened in modern medicine new doors for engaging in public understanding of science. In its incarnation in the Science Museum as *Health Matters* (now closed), it explored 'how medical technology, health surveys and medical research have changed the way we experience medicine' and showed 'how innovation and mass production have transformed medicine'.[5] Putting an 'iron lung built by car workers and a kidney machine made out of a tin can' on display, the exhibition aimed to explain how technology had changed medicine during the twentieth century. Over the century, however, medicine's prestigious objects like the 'kidney machine' exhausted their value of attraction and the target objects of medicine reached beyond the realm of the visible, posing new challenges for exhibition designers who are now facing the task of visualizing abstract and invisible entities like genetic risks. Re-opened in 2019 as *Medicine: The Wellcome Galleries*, the space is advertised as 'the magnificent new home for the most significant medical collections in the world,' but a 'contemplative gallery' employs especially commissioned works of art for exploring 'faith, hope and fear' while another focuses on personal experiences for examining 'the core purpose of medicine'.[6] Personal stories now have to make good for the miniaturization of medicine's objects and the alienation apparently intrinsic to medicine.

The zooming-in of medicine on ever smaller and more abstract entities coincided with a remarkable re-surfacing of the anatomical exhibition in popular culture, when Gunther von Hagens's *Body Worlds* of plastinated human remains in lifelike poses made headlines and travelled the world. The show, raising massive concerns because of the public display of dead bodies, celebrated a cult of the real body in times of its disappearance, but von Hagens justified it by educational intentions and the artful aesthetics of his exhibition. Indeed, the aesthetic experiences his exhibitions offered revolved around enlightening the visitor about the human body as a wonder of nature – by means of natural body parts transformed into plastic objects. The real body, though not the dead, but the living and suffering body, had already earlier proven a rich space of aesthetic exploration a generation before *Body Worlds* in the new genre of performance art. Artists like Vito Acconci, Hannah Wilke and Marina Abramović exposed the body as object and as subjective agency (Jones, 1998). Investigating on stage and public display the mundane or the painful, the repetition of bodily movements, the scars of a treatment or the decay of the diseased body, they questioned and performed subjectivity. Body art had related to the objectification of the body in radically different ways to the *Body Worlds* exhibition at a time when the human body had become questionable as a stable entity. With medicine advancing to molecular levels and into abstract constructs, new art projects started meanwhile to question these very processes by turning the art gallery into a genetics laboratory or by visualizing the chains of translation going into the construction of biomedical objects (Zylinska, 2009).

Exhibitions and health campaigns illustrate the dynamics of objectification also in another domain and direction – as commodification of behaviour. With the 'human factor' as the common cause for many preventable diseases, public health education advertised health guidelines in often unusually frank language and imagery (Serlin, 2010). A telling case is the safer sex campaign following upon the HIV pandemic. With the discovery of the virus and the ways of its transmission, the prevention of infection turned into a question of survival and gave rise to numerous campaigns. The safer sex campaigns show the complex socio-political embedding of public health initiatives. AIDS activists, for example, successfully challenged the FDA to change its drug-testing regulation, thereby pointing to the many actors involved in health politics in modern society (Epstein, 1996). After a century of political activism and consumer advocacy, medical experts and health authorities are still powerful actors, especially in alliance with health insurers and the pharmaceutical industry. Citizens, clients and patients, however, are no passive receivers of information

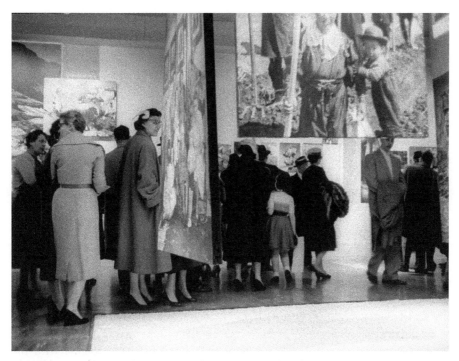

FIGURE 5.5: The Family Of Man exhibit organised by photographer Edward Steichen at the Museum of Modern Art. Credit: Michael Rougier / Contributor / Getty Images.

and guidelines. This pertains especially to the HIV epidemic where the global inequalities exacerbated as drastic discrepancies and differences in access to health care, prevention and stigmatization (Messac and Prabhu, 2013), turning AIDS into a major issue of global health and human rights (Mold and Reubi, 2013).

The visual display of the healthy body interfered with body politics in modern society on many levels. Unlike any other area of medical practice, cosmetic surgery, for example, is directly related to the discourse on the perfect body in popular culture (Harris-Moore, 2014). Cosmetic surgery thus offers insights into the societal dynamics of professional body modification unconstrained by the limits of therapeutic medicine. It offers a technological fix for the desired body shape, thereby responding to and nurturing a public demand. Here, a new mode of biopolitics becomes recognizable, driven by the feedback loops between the media, society, clients and specialists. This biopolitics is not installed from above, but mediated within society. The making available of technological solutions seizes on an economic opportunity, may respond to a need and creates a demand. For the time being, the commodification of the body appears to be the course. It finds its complement in the rise of gadgets for self-monitoring, tracking everything from food intake to the number of steps, the heart rate or the scores on a happiness scale as quantified measures. Apparently, the instruments' access to the body has meanwhile beaten bodily self-perception.

THE VIRTUALIZATION OF MEDICINE AND ITS RE-APPROPRIATION

Medicine populated the world with many objects, from tools and instruments used in its practice via natural entities like antibodies or genes to the large infrastructures for research and treatment – not to forget the many things medicine introduced into daily life like vitamins, calories or antiseptic sprays. These objects interact with the sociocultural fabric of society and the life-worlds of patients in a myriad of ways in relation to the epistemic and economic, the personal and political relevance of these objects. Medicine participated at the commodification of the human body and was a major driving force for its objectification. The objectifying gaze of medicine's visual cultures converted organic details to powerful representations of disease that were then targeted by technologized interventions. If in medicine representing and intervening have meanwhile successfully been delegated to monitoring screens and machine guided instruments, the next step will be to complement medicine with the simulation and modelling of the human body and of individual cases of diseases (Hacking, 1983). The *Visible Human Project* started this trend: preserving a human body as a data pool, the project assembled and correlated visualizations from diagnostic techniques such as CT-scanning with photographs from the dissected body (Waldby, 2000). The project not only blurred further the distinction between living and dead bodies that was initiated with the linking of clinical signs to post-mortem evidence, but also blended the two opposing meanings of 'model' as exemplar and simulation.

Today the so-called personalized medicine pushing medical practice in a similar direction. Initially advertised as an outcome of the *Human Genome Project* harvesting its results and delivering individualized health care on the basis of genetic data, personalized medicine has now been moved to the spaces of virtualization. Because the anticipated predictive powers of genetic testing crumbled in light of new insights from epigenetics, personalized medicine is currently promoted as a form of digitalized medical practice integrating all available information (Collins et al., 2001). Massively aligning genetic information with postgenomic and epigenetic data, microbiome data and clinical case histories, the precision medicine of the future will treat patients in form of large data bodies integrating all available information. Simulating the disease trajectories in relation to the available therapeutic intervention in computer models of individual patient cases, this medicine envisions custom-tailored therapies (Brown, 2015). The history of objectifying medicine that was started with the invention, construction and implementation of diagnostic technology into clinical practice some 200 years ago and which had reached its first peak with the operation of real patients on computer screens displaying representations of their diseases is now going virtual by treating patient avatars.

Contextualizing the cultural history of biomedicine's objects is such a way to a history of objectification resonates with the Marxist theory of reification and alienation. The commodification of the body in society echoes Marx' analysis of the fetish and exemplifies the consequences of the capitalist mode of production with its division of labour in the health sector (Marx, 1990: 160ff). Common complains about alienating experiences with health services may foster this argument. However, very few people would decide against treatment in cases of accident, stroke or heart attack. In a similar vein, most people would (understandably) agree with a carefully planned hip replacement, although it being an example of totally objectified surgery. Apparently objectification and alienation do not follow from each other, and objectification can become part of individual strategies of self-optimization.

If it is less the alienation part of Marx' analysis, certainly the political economy applies to objectification in medicine and especially to the objectification of the body. Objectification has become a particularly powerful mode to connect the body (and thereby the living being, such as the athletic as well as the suffering individual) to the logics of investment and exchange value. In addition to the objectification processes driven by the pharmaceutical industry and medical technology, medicine participates at the commodification of the human body itself. Just like other objects, the human body, its particular shape or specific body parts become fetishized and are fed into the market value system. According to this logic, objects represent diversions of capital that articulate in cascades of exchange value in more and more interconnected markets.

Biomedicine exhibits the capitalist powers of the commodification of the body and the pervasive penetration of the health sector by the neoliberal agenda. But objectification and commodification operates on all sides and in many different ways, integrating epistemic regimes of knowledge with politics of value and mediating unforeseen paths for appropriation by the various actors (Appadurai, 1986). Objectification is not a one-way street to alienation and the appropriation of the body for reclaiming health may rather build on the objectification of the body than result from a nostalgic flight to its allegedly undisturbed nature. Objectification appears to be a permanently ongoing, dynamic and highly productive process that is neither controlled by medicine (although it certainly is a powerful player) nor limited to its domain. As objectifying colonization of the world, biomedicine participates at larger processes, generating ever-new objects and bringing about more questions together with the problems it promises to solve. Appropriation, alienation and social mediation continue to take on new forms in the object cultures of biomedicine.

NOTES

1. This applies especially to more popular accounts of the history of medicine; see, for example, Schott (1993).
2. This transformation of medicine by diagnostic technology has been carefully studied since Stanley Reiser's seminal study (Reiser, 1981) in the history of medicine (Howell, 1996; Lachmund, 1997), but its epistemological implications have hardly been taken up by philosophy of medicine, cf. Borck (2016).
3. I am referring here especially to Friedrich Kittler and German media theory, which took the Canadian school of media studies by Harold Innis and Marshall McLuhan further by questioning the material conditions of discourse as their fundamental epistemic underpinnings, cf. Kittler (1990).
4. TIME magazine: 100 photos; the most influential images of all time, http://100photos.time.com (last accessed 10 October 2020).
5. This and the following quote are from the still existing web page of the Health Matters exhibition, cf. http://www.sciencemuseum.org.uk/visitmuseum/plan_your_visit/exhibitions/health_matters (last accessed 13 February 2017).
6. https://www.sciencemuseum.org.uk/see-and-do/medicine-wellcome-galleries (last accessed 10 October 2020) and https://learning.sciencemuseumgroup.org.uk/wp-content/uploads/2019/11/Medicine-The-Wellcome-Galleries-Gallery-Guide.pdf (last accessed 10 October 2020) for the description of thematic galleries.

CHAPTER SIX

Experience

JULIE LIVINGSTON

Biomedicine is a set of ideas and practices brought to bear on a human being. As such, it is built into a society through the embodied and emotional experiences of patients as much as through the political economy or cultural authority of its ideas, institutions and markets. The history of biomedicine, then, can be understood as a changing set of experiences. A phenomenological approach theorizes medicine in light of its putative purpose – the easing of affliction and the promotion of well-being. Holding tight to the register of feeling highlights the tensions and ambiguities so often effaced in master narratives of biomedicine and a novel cultural history emerges in the interstices. This is a history that attends to side effects and pain as much as disease, to hopes and fears as much as ideas and innovations, to access and communication as much as normative practice. Experience reveals how the body in all its excess is shaped by medicine and yet so often subverts its claims, even claims to 'patient-centred care'.

From the 1920s to the close of the twentieth century, shifting epidemiological patterns marked by the general decline of infectious disease, the rise of chronic illness, global pandemics, devastating wars and the development of an array of new medical technologies all reshaped the temporal, social, economic and phenomenological experience of biomedical care. Over the twentieth century, the reach of biomedicine was greatly extended. This was accomplished geographically first through European and North American colonial and missionary medicine, and then with the subsequent rise of international and global health institutions and programmes, premised on biomedicine. Within the global North, the reach of biomedicine extended ever further into social and political life, as a secularizing explanatory force, as a site of hope and mastery over nature, and as a set of tools through which self-making occurred.

Hospitals became important sites of safety and care for the sick as well as zones of expensive technology superseding their previous iteration as charitable institutions that primarily serviced the poor. Pharmaceutical and other medical technologies became commonplace and often part of daily rituals of self-care and maintenance. As such, in the twentieth century experiences of medicine became both quotidian and dramatic.

Yet biomedicine's increasing power and prevalence was not without its frictions. People did not experience medicine uniformly. While biomedicine has become a global system, political and economic factors distribute it unevenly. Nor do biomedical knowledge and practice stand outside of or apart from the larger culture in which they operate. In many parts of the world by the close of the twentieth century, biomedicine was still far from hegemonic. Rather it co-existed, combined and competed with other therapeutic systems. This means that the experience of medicine was caught up in power in a range of particular ways – as a site of colonial coercion, post-colonial object of desire, tool of Christian proselytization, instantiation or negation of human right or national citizenship.

Within the US, Canada, Europe and Australia, politically oppressed minorities experienced this coercive power of biomedicine through its relationship to local political economies in which they might receive poor quality care or no care at all, and to the coercive powers of medical authority that made them vulnerable to the predations of medical experimentation, and policies like eugenic sterilization. Differences of class, age, education, race, religion, sexuality, gender and disability status all shaped how patients encountered medical practice and experienced medical authority. Beginning in the 1960s, activists from various groups including feminist, queer, disabled and black sought to reshape the clinical encounter and to challenge the politics underpinning it. Their critiques exposed the political roots of the stratified and complex nature of patient experience. Their actions helped to produce changes in clinical culture.

This chapter reviews various changes in experiences of biomedicine from the 1920s to the close of the twentieth century. Medicine is a relationship and the experiences of clinicians, nurses and lay caregivers are vital, heterodox and subject to historical change. But in the interest of space, this chapter centres attention primarily on the experiences of patients, backgrounding the interlocking experiences of caregiving. The discussion focuses on a few select domains and dynamics. It begins with cardinal events in the life cycle: childbirth and dying. It then moves to discuss two significant conceptual and political and economic processes that shape experience: medical citizenship and the embodiment of risk. It concludes by looking at two twentieth-century epidemics, HIV/AIDS and cancer, which both drive and exemplify critical developments in patient experience. These examples, and the geographic sites in which they are taken up, while far from exhaustive, have been chosen to help reveal broader patterns in the experience of medicine.

MEDICALIZING BIRTH

For many women, pregnancy brought their first sustained or intensive experience of biomedicine. What had once been a female rite of passage, whose substantial dangers were managed in the home, over time, became a medical event that extended from conception to perinatal care. The twentieth century witnessed a revolution in obstetric practice, bringing birth further under medical management. From the rise of antenatal care to the refinement and marked increase of caesarean section, concerns regarding infant feeding practices, and an emphasis on the hospital as the safest site for parturition, women increasingly experienced pregnancy and motherhood through biomedical knowledge and practice. New techniques and technologies of prediction such as amniocentesis and ultrasound further shaped the experience of pregnancy as at once intimate and social, embodied and political. Such changes were felt differently across the globe at different times. So too were the process of birth and the clinical encounters that surrounded it inseparable from local norms of morality. For example, unmarried women in some times and contexts might find themselves shamed, punished or shunned by clinical staff, thus folding the physical and social discomforts of childbirth together.

In the United States and Canada, the period between 1880 and 1920 saw the consolidation of medical authority over obstetrics, setting the stage for the increasing medicalization of pregnancy and childbirth (Leavitt, 1987; Mitchinson, 2002). From the 1920s onwards, certain patterns emerged over the course of the century that shaped normative experiences of pregnancy and childbirth. These patterns included a precipitous drop in the risk of maternal death; the move from home to hospital births; and the array of technologies from amniocentesis to ultrasound to the foetal heart monitor that rendered the foetus an object of medical observation. Such developments were also played out across much of the global North, though not uniformly. For example, Sweden and the Netherlands already by the 1920s had low rates of maternal mortality, and by the end of the century approximately thirty per cent of Dutch women still delivered their babies at home (Marland, 2000). Meanwhile, within the US, urban women made the move to hospital deliveries before their rural counterparts.

Childbirth had long been a profoundly dangerous process, one that women both feared and respected. With improvements in nutrition and basic health, antiseptic knowledge and practice, blood transfusion and eventually antibiotics, maternal mortality rates began to fall in much of the global North. Yet if women experienced medicalization in part as an easing of their fears of dying, they also experienced hospital-based deliveries as routinized and alienating. Women, who began entering hospital maternity wards in large numbers in the 1930s and 1940s could expect to be sedated with analgesics, draped, laid on a table and put into stirrups. Thus the experience of giving birth had become quasi-surgical.

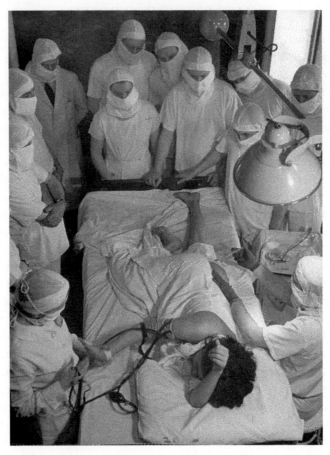

FIGURE 6.1: Operating room staff (doctors, nurses, etc., all w. masks) watching as anesthesiologist gives woman about to deliver a baby an epidural injection during painless childbirth at the Lying In Hospital. Credit: Alfred Eisenstaedt / Contributor / Getty Images.

They would deliver in the lithotomy position. Gone were the array of positions and the ability to transition between them that women had utilized while giving birth at home. By the 1940s and 1950s, they could expect to be shaved, receive an enema, have contractions induced with Pitocin and have their perineal opening cut painfully deep into the muscular tissue with scissors all at the (almost invariably male) doctor's direction. To give birth in hospital meant the surrender of one's body to the institution, which reworked the pain of labour into new configurations.

Perhaps the most disorienting and profound change that medicalization brought to labouring women was the experience of giving birth alone. As the site of delivery moved from home to hospital, women no longer spent their labouring hours surrounded by female relatives and neighbours. US historian Judith Leavitt quotes women from the late 1930s through to the late 1950s on this experience of isolation:

> 'The cruelest part of [hospital] childbirth is being alone among strangers,' wrote one woman . . . Others remembered being 'all alone', 'abandoned', and 'lonely . . . knowing no one'. The *Ladies' Home Journal* revealed some of the fault lines in its 1958 exposé. One woman wrote about her experiences in a suburban hospital outside Chicago: 'I wonder if the people who ran that place were actually human. My lips parched and cracked, but the nurses refused to even moisten them with a damp cloth. I was left alone all night in a labor room. I felt exactly like a trapped animal . . . Never have I needed someone, anyone, as desperately as I did that night.' Another woman wrote, 'I remember screaming, "help me, help me!" to a nurse who was sitting at a nearby desk. She ignored me.
>
> —Leavitt, 2009: 34–9

As hospital-based delivery expanded globally, the experience of social isolation became one of its defining characteristics from mid-century Britain to post-Soviet Russia (King, 2016; Rivkin-Fish, 2000). Within the global South, the move to the hospital came later and was incomplete. Yet the experience of isolation, the lithotomy position and giving over to the authority of clinical staff resonate, though analgesics were not on offer. Consider the following example recorded by anthropologist Liv Haram in the mid-1980s in the southern African nation of Botswana:

> Miss J is admitted to the labour room. Her cervical os is 8 cm dilated and she is having painful contractions. She is restless, turning from side to side and groaning loudly. She is searching for support with her hands on the headboard of the bed . . . The door to the corridor is wide open. There is no midwife in the labour room. An orderly comes in, looks around and walks out again. It seems that Miss J. is pushing.
>
> At 9:30 Miss J. is uttering words of pain and becomes more restless. At 9:40 midwife A comes in and writes on the labour graph of Miss J. that she didn't bring her antenatal clinic card. She looks at Miss J. and tells her not to push and that she will be there to deliver her: 'In the hospital nobody delivers by herself.' She repeats this while leaving the labour room.
>
> —Anderson and Staugart, 1986: 58

Beginning in the mid-1960s, as part of the feminist health movement in the US and Western Europe, women began to push back against this isolation and to bring about a shift in gender norms as they agitated to bring expectant fathers into the delivery room. By the 1980s, the presence of these fathers had become normal and expected. But many women also bristled at male and paternalistic control of birth. The women's health movement brought a new vision of 'natural childbirth', doing away with the drugs and procedures like episiotomy that had become standard. Yet this vision co-existed with a steady rise in rates of caesarean section, particularly in Latin America and North America (Betran et al., 2016). By the end of the century, for many women, the experience of delivering a child had become a surgical one.

This period also saw the development of new forms of birth control that gave women (and in some cases men) new ways of controlling their fertility. For many women, access to new forms of birth control changed their experience of sexuality by delinking it to pregnancy, and of their bodies by, for example, regulating or altering their menstrual cycles. For some poor, black, brown and disabled women, these new techniques and technologies might mean unwanted sterilization. This process built on the extensive eugenic policies of American state of California and, most infamously, Nazi Germany, which sterilized some 400,000 people (Proctor, 1988). In post-Second World War Puerto Rico, and apartheid-era Namibia, for example, women might awake from caesarean section without realizing the doctor had also performed a tubal ligation. These women joined the many others from India to China to the United States who were compelled by the state to undergo surgical sterilization or to accept the insertion of an IUD (Lindsay, 1991; Schoen, 2005; Rodriguez-Trias, 1978; Lopez, 1993; Connolly, 2006). Such compulsions worked through carrots as well as sticks. For example, from the 1950s to the 1970s in India, financial incentives were offered to women who accepted IUDs and men who underwent vasectomy. The programme was later replaced by a less coercive one, which still provided financial incentives for women's tubal ligation in addition to men's vasectomy. Thus biomedical techniques and practices were part of a novel experience in which a person's fertility might be commodified in contexts of pervasive hunger and poverty (Gwatkin, 1979; Singh et al., 2012). They were also at the centre of expansive feelings of sorrow not only by some women and men who experienced negative physical effects of these procedures, but also by many who regretted the loss of their fertility.

Ironically, 'natural' childbirth, though less paternalistic, was still a medicalized experience. This was because pregnancy itself had become a protracted medical event, of which parturition was only one element. Beginning in the 1940s, antenatal care, with its attendant recommendations about diet and behaviour, became an increasingly normative part of pregnancy for women in the global North, a process that subsequently expanded (albeit unevenly) through the South as a desired norm. By the 1980s, sonography had become a standard technological rite during the second trimester of pregnancy, and amniocentesis entered into widespread use among women deemed at higher risk for a range of inherited conditions. The embodied and imaginative experiences of pregnancy were increasingly routed through technologies of visualization that figured the interior of the female body and that of the gestating foetus. As medical anthropologist Rayna Rapp suggests, predictive technologies like amniocentesis turned pregnant women into 'moral pioneers' who faced personal bioethical decisions about disability and abortion (Rapp, 1999). By the opening of the twenty-first century, amid high rates of congenital malformations brought by the toxic legacy of the US military's widespread use of dioxin and other chemicals, many pregnant women in Vietnam along with their partners sought out repeated ultrasounds. Many then experienced, in conversation with kin, difficult bioethical decisions about pregnancy termination (Gammeltof, 2014).

MEDICALIZING DEATH

In many parts of the global North over the course of the twentieth century, death, much like birth, increasingly became a biomedical process and as such the experience of dying would change significantly. As with birth, the medicalization of death over time also produced a backlash. Nurses and doctors with the support of patients eventually developed a philosophy stressing the value of care at the end of life, which resulted in a more 'natural', less high-tech site for dying, the hospice, while other patients died in their homes supported by the care of a visiting hospice nurse. But as with birth, by this time more 'natural' forms of dying were already shaped by biomedicine.

The medicalization of death in Europe, North America, Japan and Australia actually began in the nineteenth century. But by the 1920s, throughout the global North most people would still expect to die in their homes among family members, albeit under a doctor's care, thus making death a solemn and intimate, religious, yet familiar experience for many. By the end of the twentieth century, the hospital had become the normative locus for dying. The gradual extension of life expectancy in the global North, combined with demographic changes in the proportion of elderly people, and epidemiological changes manifest in the rise in chronic terminal illness, meant that the medical experience of dying was increasingly (though by no means exclusively) a protracted one.

In the early decades of the twentieth century, doctors were already often providing morphine to the dying. Dying was often still quite painful, but the pain was now experienced and understood as a technical phenomenon as much as a moral or spiritual one, and the power of palliation was tightly held by the doctor. Beginning in the 1960s, the nascent hospice movement began in the UK by articulating a model of pain-management versus pain relief, and the fuzzy rush of opioid analgesics followed by the easing of pain became increasingly central to the experience of dying. The temporality of dying was now partially

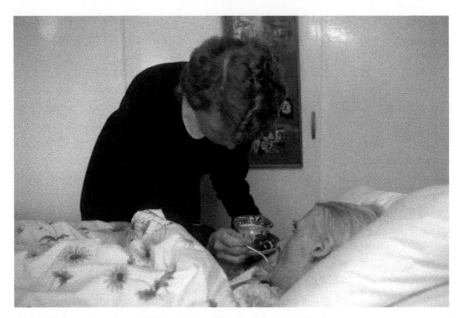

FIGURE 6.2: NHS District nurse caring for a dying woman at home. Credit: Sally
and Richard Greenhill / Alamy Stock Photo.

driven by the clock, as patients wracked with pain awaited their next scheduled
dose of morphine. Soon morphine pumps were developed so that dying patients
lying in hospital could squeeze a button and control pain on command. For
many, this meant that death was preceded by opioid-induced dreamy moving in
and out of consciousness. Unfortunately for some patients, as they neared the
end of protracted dying experiences, such opioids failed to produce relief any
longer.

With hospitalization and intensifying medical management, by the 1960s
the phenomenology of dying was elaborated in new ways. Pneumonia was
once called the 'old person's friend' for the way in which it eased frail elderly
people to a quiet death. By the 1970s, elderly patients with pneumonia would
increasingly be brought to hospital and stabilized with antibiotics, intravenous
rehydration fluids and other supports, then returned home or to a long-term
residential care facility. Thus the spiral towards death became cyclical for some
patients. Amid cyclical patterns of crisis, patients also lingered with escalating
bodily experiences like dyspnoea (shortness of breath). Tethered to oxygen
tanks, one could gasp for months in the technologically diffused panic of a
slow-motion death.

New technologies developed in response to the devastating global polio
pandemics of the late 1940s and early 1950s saw the birth of the intensive
care unit. The first unit was developed in Denmark to provide individual

round-the-clock care to acute polio patients who required respiratory assistance (Kelly et al., 2014). As intensive medicine grew and spread, the mechanical (and eventually computerized) respirator would become the cornerstone of the ICU, allowing new forms of dying to emerge. The ICU became the destination of those critically injured in the new epidemic of road accidents, and in the United States, gunshots, alongside those who had suffered severe heart attacks, stroke, organ failure or the pneumonia of the dying. Mechanical breathing confined patients to their beds. It also required intubation – the placing of a breathing tube into the airway either through the mouth, which prevents patients from speaking, or via a tracheostomy. In either case, patients on respirators were often heavily sedated, sometimes comatose, hydrated intravenously, and fed through a tube and catheterized. For those who were conscious, intubation might bring panic and frustration. ICUs became technologically dense sites where patients were connected to various monitors and webs of intravenous tubing, and supported by nurses who cared for patients often via machine. This was a new and surreal experience of the body extended through the machine. The nurses who worked in the ICU had to address this humanity of the person in this surreal body and the profound alienation and anxiety of the patient's loved ones, while directing their attention to complex challenges of multiple machines, networks of tubing and electrical cords, and carefully timed medications and procedures.

By the end of the century, some technologies of the ICU had become internalized, thereby extending the dying process in ways that would become widespread in the twenty-first century. The implantable pacemaker had become standard therapy for cardiac patients whose hearts required electrical stimulation to maintain regular rhythm. By the end of the twentieth century, many pacemakers were now fitted with internal cardiac defibrillators, which are programmed to detect lethal rhythms and then shock the heart back into regular rhythm. Such technologies are implantable versions of the hospital defibrillator machine, which is standard equipment in both trauma and intensive care units. The painful, unpredictable shock of the defibrillator now internalized is experienced as both tremendously aversive and yet also lifesaving (Kaufman et al., 2011).

By the late 1960s, life-support technologies originally forged in the ICU further enabled entirely new phenomenological possibilities – the persistent vegetative state, and brain death. In these states, patients are warm to the touch, they can continue to produce tears and spontaneous physical movements, but are completely unconscious. The person in the persistent vegetative state has brain activity and possibly some form of sentience, as well as the potential for the recovery of consciousness and bodily function, while the brain-dead 'neo-mort' does not. Brain death, as anthropologist Margaret Lock has explained, was a new category of death determined by experts in the US. It emerged in relation to the new surgical possibilities for solid organ transplants and was taken up as a defined form of death at different times in different countries. Americans and Canadians accepted this new form of hybrid experience as death in the 1970s, while Danes did not accept this designation until the early 1990s, and the high-tech pioneering Japanese and Koreans debated it yet longer (Lock, 2001).

Meanwhile, the experience of organ transfer that brain death facilitates raised philosophical and existential questions about biomedical experience, and its locus within the body. Many recipients of solid organs from 'living cadavers' reported profound feelings around the intimate incorporation of a vital element of another person within their body, sometimes manifest in new and surprising gustatory desires or emotional states (Sharp, 2006). The commodification of bodily parts, experienced by Indian women exchanging functioning fallopian tubes for badly needed cash, would soon be mirrored by a global black market in human organs that transferred kidneys, eye globes and other tissue from putatively healthy poor sellers to wealthy but ailing buyers via profit-making brokers (Scheper Hughes, 2006; Cohen, 1999). In this new techno-medical landscape, some came to experience their bodies as partible, and thereby as an economic resource of last resort.

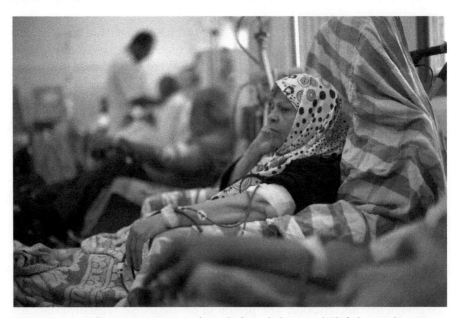

FIGURE 6.3: Palestinian patients undergo kidney dialysis at al-Shifa hospital in Gaza City on September 14, 2013. The health situation in the Gaza Strip faces difficulties since the closure of the Rafah crossing which has prevented the entry of Egyptian fuel into the Strip and the flow of some 1,000 patients a month requiring medical care in Egypt. Credit: MAHMUD HAMS / Staff / Getty Images.

EMBODYING RISK

One of the most profound developments in the second half of the twentieth century was a reorientation of the relationship between somatic experience and patient subjectivity. This period witnessed what historian/clinician Robert Aronowitz calls 'the converged experience of risk and disease' (Aronowitz, 2009). As new and ever more sensitive screening technologies met with new pharmaceutical and medical device strategies around the treatment of biological markers, patients in the global North became caught up in 'diagnosis creep'. In this way, people without any physical symptoms of illness began to understand themselves as patients and to undertake biomedical projects in accordance with this understanding. As Aronowitz puts it:

> The experience of being at risk for disease is not only a psychological response to the probabilities of this or that outcome. It is also constituted by predictable and structured routines, resulting in a characteristic risk experience or state. This *risk state* may be similar to the experience of a bona fide disease. Risk is often embodied, adding to its disease-ness.
>
> —Aronowitz, 2005: 49

One of the earliest and best examples of this process is the rise of risk factors in relation to heart disease. Whereas in the early decades of the twentieth century, medical wisdom held coronary heart disease to be a degenerative condition, by mid-century this reasoning, underscored in relation to the massive Framingham heart study, gave way to the idea that heart disease was the product of multiple risk factors. In the United States, amid rising rates of heart disease, people who experienced no symptoms of illness began to find themselves as proto-patients cautioned that they were prone to dropping dead suddenly. This was determined by a steady proliferation of risk factors such as gender (male), blood pressure, smoking history, cholesterol levels and family history. Historian Jeremy Greene has documented how the pharmaceutical industry took up the new paradigm of multiple interacting risk factors as the basis for a new business model in which preventive medicine would be pharmaceuticalized. In the process, people were encouraged to know their cholesterol levels and their blood pressure, such knowledge underscoring their need to ingest daily doses of diuretics, statins and/or beta blockers. Thus by the final decades of the twentieth century, millions of Americans regularly consumed drugs for conditions that produced no physical symptoms, even as the drugs themselves might produce palpable side effects (Greene, 2008).

Genetic screening is one of the emergent areas in which the risk paradigm has grown. Notions of hereditary disease were long-standing, to which the history of eugenic sterilizations and amniocentesis discussed earlier attests. By the final decade of the twentieth century, genetic screening technology had progressed from amniocentesis for high-risk pregnancies to the identification of probabilistic genetic risk for later disease expression among asymptomatic adults. For example, women might undergo genetic testing to identify through the presence of genetic mutations BRCA1 or BRCA2 that put them at substantially higher risk for breast cancer and ovarian cancer syndrome. The confirmed presence of BRCA1 or BRCA2 in turn resituates the experience of the body and of risk. Women in this situation exist in a state of anxious, pre-symptomatic patienthood, undergoing more regular monitoring for the presence of cancer. In perhaps the most extreme example of the convergence of risk and disease, some women find existing in a state of 'high-risk' dangerous or stressful enough that they undergo voluntary prophylactic breast amputation, surgically removing healthy breast tissue that is already experienced as future disease. Sociologists Carlos Novas and Nikolas Rose's observation in relation to genetic screening can be fruitfully extended to the risk paradigm more broadly, 're-cataloguing illness and pathologies along a genetic axis does not generate fatalism. On the contrary it creates an obligation to act in the present in relation to the potential futures that now come into view' (Novas and Rose, 2000: 486).

EXPERIENCING CITIZENSHIP

Medical experience is also political experience. Sometimes this fact is invisible, submerged deep below the level of consciousness; at other times it is an explicit, palpable aspect of experience. In the twentieth century, this has been made apparent through popular resistance to public health programmes that compel adherence, like vaccination or sterilization campaigns. Increasingly over the twentieth century, medicine also came to function as a gateway or adjudicating mechanism through which people were deemed deserving of other social services or supports. In such contexts experiences of medicine citizenship in terms of political claims might be experienced through biological status that requires medical authority. As Adriana Petryna explains in her work on biological citizenship, after the breakup of the Soviet Union, people in Ukraine whose suffering was determined to be a result of radiation exposure to the recent Chernobyl nuclear disaster qualified for crucial government services and compensation. In such a context, patients struggled to get doctors to certify them, their medical experiences now the only vehicle for state support (Petryna, 2003). Doctors and nurses, in turn, felt conflicted and disheartened in their roles as gatekeepers and resource-brokers, managing access to a zero-sum game of limited resources amid widespread need.

In contexts where the state provides biomedical care, medicine, in all its complexity, can be experienced as a manifestation of citizenship. Errors or alienation at the hospital become errors of or alienation by the state, while

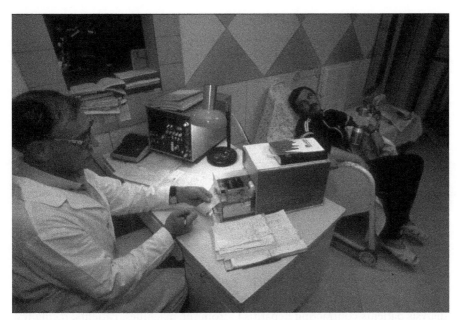

FIGURE 6.4: Man who worked at Chernobyl nuclear plant at time of 1986 radiation-releasing accident having background radiation in his body checked at Chernobyl workers health clinic where workers live for 1 month each year. January 01, 1990. Credit: Chuck Nacke / Contributor / Getty Images.

successes and care at the hospital becomes care by the state. As the state changed, so did medicine. For example, after Britain established its National Health Service in 1948, British people began to receive the vast majority of their medical care as a right of citizenship. As historian Alex Mold has suggested, in the ensuing decades Britons seeking care through the NHS increasingly experienced medical subjectivity at the unstable intersection of a triple identity: patient, consumer, citizen (Mold, 2012).

From the 1950s to the 1970s, many southern countries attempted to build state health services out of the patchwork of colonial medical institutions they had inherited at independence. In perhaps the most famous case, Cuba, this form of medical citizenship began at the revolution in 1959 and was subsequently developed through services like the polyclinics opened in 1965 and enshrined as a constitutional right by 1976. The growing cadre of community-based doctors and nurses who staffed the national medical service were envisioned and encountered as extensions of the revolution. The intimacy of the medical encounter for better or for worse was a political intimacy as well.

Yet beginning in the 1980s at the behest of creditors like the Bretton Woods Institutions (the World Bank and the International Monetary Fund), and then accelerating after the collapse of the Soviet Union, in many places health services were gradually privatized, hollowed out and increasingly iatrogenic. As a result, by the final decades of the century many patients experienced biomedicine as an extension of the frustrating bureaucratic power of the state married to the hollowness or partiality of its promises, while an imagined, idealized, efficacious biomedicine remained out of reach, the purview of the rich and powerful. In Cuba this began in the 1990s as shortages of medicines and supplies accompanied a precipitous drop in the number of surgeries performed. By the end of the decade, for many Cubans a visit to the hospital became an occasion to critique the state (Brotherton, 2005).

Anthropologist Sherine Hamdy describes a situation in Egypt at the end of the twentieth century where amid high rates of kidney disease, low-income patients must spend hours each week tethered to dialysis machines for 'blood washing'. 'Many of the patients had been misdiagnosed and mistreated prior to complete loss of kidney function. Some patients were prescribed the wrong medication, leading to acute kidney failure; others lost kidney function after botched operations for removal of kidney stones' (Hamdy, 2008: 558). Dialysis itself was in turn iatrogenic, with an estimated seventy to eight per cent of dialysis patients contracting hepatitis C from the machines. Patients, facing few options, experienced the failure of medicine and the failure of the state as a single phenomenon. As Hamdy explains,

> Patients suffer not only from the disease itself but also from inferior treatment: Their intense ambivalence toward medicalization is evident in their utter dependence on the very state provision of services that they fear could further harm them. Dialysis patients are literally connected to machines that are themselves connected to state infrastructure and its not always reliable delivery of skills, labor, and power.
>
> —Hamdy, 2006: 556

Such examples, which are not limited to the global South, further reveal how experiences of biomedical technologies are always historically contextual. When dialysis machines appeared in select hospitals in the early 1960s, US patients competed for access to the miraculous new life-saving machines. Dialysis was always physically exhausting, required being stuck with needles, and often caused leg cramps and other side effects. But in the 1960s it was also an experience that was saturated with uncertainty. Patients did not know how long their lives could be extended with this new technology. With the development of kidney transplant in the following decades, and the refinement of dialysis technology and knowledge, the experience of being tethered to the machine shifted. While exhaustion, leg cramps and other physical experiences continued to mark dialysis treatment, uncertainty now coalesced around hope for transplantation and organ waiting lists. Dialysis once experienced as miraculous was now a necessary, yet burdensome placeholder. For those patients in contexts where equipment was old and poorly maintained, and where electricity supply was uneven and prone to failure, added layers of doubt and anxiety contributed to the burden.

CANCER

Cancer was already a feared affliction in many parts of the world by the 1920s. But over the subsequent decades its prevalence would slowly, inexorably grow until by the turn of the twenty-first century, epidemiologists estimated a global population of more than 24 million cancer patients (Parkin et al., 2005). In the early decades of the century, doctors treated cancers either with surgery or with new radiation technologies. By the 1940s, the first chemotherapeutic agents were put into use and the post-Second World War era saw the birth and development of oncology as a medical sub-speciality. Experiences of oncology highlighted the fact that biomedical therapeutics could be brutal and arduous and that biomedical research required human subjects. As such, oncology required patient docility manifest in compulsory optimism and deference, such that the assaults of toxic, aggressive therapies could be experienced as signs of hope. For doctors whose daily work produced suffering in the name of healing, such hope was equally necessary to the task at hand. Cancer therefore provides one site for understanding the complex interplay between despair and hope, side effects and palliation that structured many experiences of biomedicine over the twentieth century.

Cancer therapies entailed a heroic ethos that harkened back to an earlier era of medical practice. Disfiguring surgeries, cytotoxic drugs and radiation treatments matched the aggression of the disease with equally aggressive interventions. Though each of these domains of oncology would be refined over the course of the century, they nonetheless made for profoundly aversive patient experiences. The late poet Lucy Greely vividly describes her first chemotherapy injection for Ewing's sarcoma in the 1970s in her memoir: 'It was an anatomy lesson. I had never known it was possible to *feel* your organs the way you feel your tongue in your mouth, or your teeth . . .' She continues with vivid, agonizing description of the violent vomiting that ensued until 'Gradually the waves of vomiting subsided, leaving behind an un-acted upon nausea that seemed to involve not just my stomach but all of me, even my feet, my scalp' (Greely, 1994: 66–7). This nausea would persist for several days before giving way. Like most chemotherapy, such treatment was given multiple times, and the pattern of nausea thus repeated itself every few weeks for some time. Cyclical time is critical to the embodied knowledge through which patients come to experience oncology (Bluebond-Langner, 1978; Livingston, 2012).

Surgeries were equally aggressive. By the 1920s, Halsted's radical mastectomy was already the standard treatment for breast cancers. This 'radical' surgery removed the breast in which a malignancy was found, as well as surrounding tissue, the axillary lymph nodes and the pectoral muscles. Women emerged from surgery debilitated and disfigured. Until the 1960s, women with suspected breast cancers experienced the gendered nature of medical paternalism through the assumption that they give over bodily autonomy to their surgeons. Women who came to the surgeon with a lump received a biopsy under anaesthesia. If the biopsy confirmed a malignancy then the radical mastectomy was performed on the spot without discussion with the patient (Lerner, 2002).

That patients gave themselves over to such aversive therapies speaks to the deep fear that cancer held for many amid its rising prevalence. For much of the twentieth century, cancer was a private experience, perhaps even one tinged with shame. It was also an intensely painful illness, one that could produce rot and stink, and one that patients recognized as likely to be fatal. In such a context, aggressive therapies, while awful, could nonetheless (at least in hindsight) be experienced as relief, when rotting tissue was excised or painful tumours shrank through radiation and chemotherapy. Patients were encouraged to wear wigs and prostheses to mask the disfiguring effects of oncology, and then expected to get on with their lives. Yet for many patients, cancer's recurrence in the years following their initial treatment would renew their desperation and dread as they faced death a second and often final time.

By the 1960s, many women patients in the US had begun to resent the paternalism they faced, and to question medical authority amid continuing high rates of cancer mortality. European and Canadian surgeons began to abandon the Halsted radical mastectomy for less radical alternatives, and in the 1970s American women eventually succeeded in pressuring US oncologists to follow suit. Yet as Audre Lorde, Barbara Ehrenreich and others have noted, by the 1980s a new breast cancer culture had emerged that rendered patients as 'survivors' and called for a compulsory optimism. Amid new therapies and a turn to patient 'autonomy' came new and subtle pressures to be 'positive' in the face of disease (Ehrenreich, 2001; Lorde, 1980). That optimism would be reinvested in oncology. The end of the Halsted procedure did not mean the end of aggressive therapy for cancer. Oncologists learned how to cure some cancers. Important successes included effective cures for much childhood leukaemia, Hodgkin's lymphoma and testicular cancer. Yet with ever-rising rates of cancer, amid relatively stable mortality rates for most cancers the American public was encouraged to invest its hopes in biomedical progress, such that patients often competed at the end of their lives to become experimental subjects in early phase clinical trials for new drugs and therapies.

Meanwhile, in response to cancer and to cancer activists, new forms of palliation and clinical communication around prognosis and treatment options would be developed in some parts of the global North. By the end of the century, new anti-emetics would help attenuate the profound nausea that chemotherapy often entailed, while morphine pumps and other analgesics (as discussed earlier) eased the tremendous pain of disease and the side effects of treatment. Yet members of racial minorities and incarcerated patients would inevitably have a harder time accessing such palliatives, despite the profound pain of their cancers (Cleeland et al., 1994; Lin and Mathew, 2005). Yet by the end of the century as patients in India, China, Kenya, and other sites in the global South began accessing oncology, they would find the aversive oncological therapies on offer without the new palliative technologies meant to soften the brutality of disease (Human Rights Watch, 2009; 2010; Krakauer, 2008).

Though cancer mortality rates remained high, over the century the trajectory of illness expanded, as new diagnostic technologies allowed for earlier detection of cancers, and as new therapies allowed some patients to live longer after diagnosis. Early detection would mean that many people became cancer patients at an earlier, and often asymptomatic, stage in their disease – new therapies that allowed patients to enter disease remission. But the uncertain dividing line between remission and cure meant that even asymptomatic patients in the aftermath of oncology found themselves 'living in prognosis', to use cancer scholar Lochlann Jain's apt term for the state of hyperawareness and dread that characterized this state of being (Jain, 2007).

HIV/AIDS

Biomedical optimism did not begin with oncology. The middle decades of the twentieth century offered increasing confidence by many in the ability of biomedicine to control infectious disease. The arrival of antibiotics beginning first in much of Europe and the US in the 1940s altered the experience of fever, of lacerations, of painful urination and other such signs. Such sensations had previously been potential pathways to abscess, sterility and even death and were endured amid palpable dread and uncertainty. But increasingly they became signs of the need for pharmaceutical intervention, and hope and then eventually a taken-for-granted sort of confidence began to accrue around antibiotics. Similarly the gradual development and dissemination of vaccines, particularly the polio vaccines of the 1950s and the global eradication of smallpox in the late 1970s, fitted into a biomedical narrative of human victory over microbes.[1] These experiences were different in the global North, where antibiotics were easily available, compared to parts of the South where access was patchier, where patient purchasing capacity might only allow for a partial course of drugs, and where in the wake of 1980s structural adjustment (privatization and economic restructuring imposed by the Bretton Woods Institutions), a surfeit of expired and counterfeit drugs joined the erosion of diagnostic testing capacity to undermine efficacy (Peterson, 2014; Okeke, 2011). By the 1990s, a patient in Conakry might experience taking antibiotics as a lottery and thereby necessarily only one approach within a plural therapeutic landscape saturated with peril and uncertainty.

Even in the North by the early 1980s, this confidence would be swiftly undermined by the emergence of a massive, mysterious and deadly pandemic of what would eventually be recognized as HIV/AIDS. This novel disease and the response to it would underscore the intimate and political nature of medical experience as well as the fragile nature of medical progress. Epidemics as many scholars have noted, are unique historical events. They serve as a magnifying lens through which the social, political, economic, intellectual and cultural relationships of a given society are rendered in vivid detail. At the same time they are engines of change, leaving society transformed in their wake (Rosenberg, 1992). The global pandemic of HIV/AIDS in the final quarter of the twentieth century therefore holds tremendous interest for the historian of experience. In its unfolding, the fault lines of race, citizenship, sexuality, class and gender were revealed, while in response to its challenges, the fields of medicine and public health were reworked in critical ways.

Epidemics are also by definition unsettling and can produce panic and blame (Rosenberg, 1992). This process is heightened by the uncertainty that surrounds emerging illnesses like AIDS, whose definitions and biological characteristics were only gradually determined over time. On the one hand, biomedical explanation for somatic phenomena legitimizes the experience of illness and potentially maps strategies for relief and containment. This can be seen clearly in the second half of the twentieth century in the United States as various groups of patients have sought medical validation and explanation for their somatic experience – from Gulf War Syndrome and Post Traumatic Stress Disorder to Sick Building Syndrome and Fibromyalgia., Diagnosis offers legitimation of what sociologists call the sick role, pushing back against suspicions of malingering and potentially unlocking resources for care. On the other hand, such diagnoses in the absence of detailed etiological understanding can serve potentially to pathologize entire classes of people, such as military veterans.

In the early years of AIDS in the United States, which were marked by the lack of biomedical understanding of this novel disease, this form of pathologization was ascribed to four groups of people: homosexual men, Haitians, haemophiliacs and heroin addicts. In this context, the biomedical establishment married their own cultural ignorance to their lack of understanding of AIDS aetiology, and thereby became a vehicle for experiences of rampant discrimination and shunning. Many patients and their allies responded through novel forms of patient activism, forging new politics and new norms in clinical research and public health. In Africa, beginning in Central Africa, and then spreading to the east and southern regions of the continent, as AIDS cases mounted, people struggled to cope with the emerging epidemic amid frank scepticism by many in biomedical aetiology. Europeans had pathologized African sexuality for centuries, and had also engaged in iatrogenic medical campaigns and practices. AIDS was a devastating experience, but its biomedicalization was uneven.

By 1983 the HIV virus had been discovered, and by 1985 a test had been established for its presence in the body, and soon processes of transmission clarified. Yet for HIV-positive persons themselves, this meant one could live as a time bomb. Testing yielded two dimensions of embodied risk. On the one hand, those asymptomatic people who tested positive now lived in anticipation of imminent prolonged and deadly illness. On the other hand, they now understood themselves to be a potential danger to their sexual and/or injecting partners and, in the case of pregnant women, their foetuses. The idea of silent infection had been around since Mary Mallon was infamously identified with typhoid in the first decade of the twentieth century. But now this designation was widespread and heavily stigmatized.

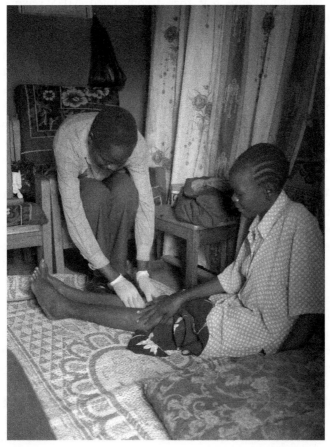

FIGURE 6.5: Comboni volunteer visiting a woman sick with AIDS, Uganda. Credit: Sean Sprague / Alamy Stock Photo.

The experience of AIDS itself was awful and disorienting. The disintegration of the body was agonizing in its unfolding and protracted in its arc. Even for patients who may have had reason to be suspicious of biomedicine, they nonetheless turned to it in extremis. Yet they ran hard up against the decided limits of biomedicine. Doctors and nurses addressed symptoms, and opportunistic infections empirically; they palliated, but could not cure. Yet biomedical palliation, which eased suffering and could prolong life, was hard to access. Many doctors and nurses, fearing the disease – a fear they might rationalize by their moral distaste for gay or drug using patients – shunned those with AIDS. In the mid-1980s, nephrologist Neil Schram was the only doctor out of 2,000 employed by Los Angeles's Kaiser Permanente to accept referrals for patients diagnosed with HIV (Bayer and Oppenheimer, 2002: 103). Even severely ill patients already admitted to hospital might find that many members of staff actively avoided them.

Meanwhile, the intense fear that accompanied AIDS reworked clinical norms. Though disposable latex gloves had been in use during invasive procedures for a decade or two, with the onset of the AIDS epidemic, doctors and nurses began wearing gloves any time they came in physical contact with a patient, reworking of the intimacy of touch in medicine. By the mid-1980s, spurred by the AIDS epidemic, so-called 'universal precautions' – gloves, masks, plastic aprons along with protocols around the disposal of needles – became standard in clinical interactions with any patient where contact with bodily fluids was possible. For patients in many parts of southern and east Africa, gloves and disposable needles, while recommended, were not always available as health budgets were eviscerated through structural adjustment imposed by Bretton Woods, and as the scale of the epidemic overwhelmed resources. By the 1990s, in some places government or NGO programmes designed to support home-based care supplied gloves and plastic sheeting, albeit intermittently, to family members who cared for AIDS patients at home. In the process, lay care practices became biomedicalized, even as many caregivers and patients alike regretted the alienation that gloves introduced into intimate practices of care.

By the mid-1990s, the first effective antiretroviral combinations had been approved for use, thus potentially altering the experience of HIV from a fatal to a chronic illness. Globally, in the final years of the twentieth century, the experience of HIV reflected new struggles over and possibilities for medical citizenship. In Brazil, for example, in 1997 the government began provision of antiretrovirals to registered AIDS cases (at the time numbering more than 100,000), while in South Africa, by 1998 that government was entering into a period of AIDS denialism, which kept the new drugs out of reach. For most of the tens of millions of infected persons who lived in sub-Saharan Africa, such expensive yet life-saving drugs remained inaccessible. Wealthy Africans and those able to access metropolitan supplies through personal contacts began taking the drugs, while for most patients on the continent the experience of HIV/AIDS was thereby politicized in new ways, extending from well-established experiences of global inequity, racism and neocolonialism. As some NGOs began small pilot programmes offering the drugs, patients were forced to scramble and compete across an uncertain archipelago of access (Nguyen, 2010; Reynolds Whyte, 2014). The arrival of the first national antiretroviral programmes in Africa and the subsequent rendering of HIV as a chronic illness would have to wait until the twenty-first century.

CONCLUSION

From 1920 to the close of the twentieth century, experiences of biomedicine underwent a set of linked changes. Formerly private experiences of birth and death increasingly moved out of the home and into the hospital. In the process, the phenomenology of pregnancy, parturition and dying shifted in the face of new forms of institutionalization and technological intervention. In the process, 'natural' became a romantic ideal against which biomedical experience was evaluated. Meanwhile the timeline of such experiences, like those of illness itself expanded as chronic illness, and the converged experience of risk and disease extended the temporality of biomedicalization, such that asymptomatic patienthood could become a long-term mode of existence. Meanwhile, the unequal distribution of medicine and the hierarchical and potentially coercive nature of biomedical care made experiences of medicine overtly political for many.

NOTE

1. This narrative was uneven and resistance to vaccination has continued from the nineteenth century until the twenty-first in various contexts. See, for example, Durbach's *Bodily Matters: The Anti-Vaccination Movement in England, 1853–1907*; Leach and Fairhead's *Vaccine Anxieties: Global Science, Child Health, and Society*; and Yahya's 'Polio vaccines – "no thank you!" Barriers to polio eradication in northern Nigeria'.

CHAPTER SEVEN

Mind and Brain

RHODRI HAYWARD

The mind and brain sciences make their own histories, although these are histories that most academic historians would struggle to recognize. The different understandings of the psyche and the nervous system that have emerged across the twentieth and twenty-first centuries contain within themselves particular projections of the past and the future: projections that appear quite bewildering to those who still persist in humanities research. This chapter does not dwell on the tensions between the neurosciences and the humanities: that subject has been explored many times and with passionate intensity (Tallis, 2010; Gopnik, 2013; Newman, 2017). Instead it attempts to recover the life-worlds that have been opened up by medical and scientific work and the new forms of practical action and political judgement that these have made possible. I trace in turn the different temporalities that have been sustained by the mind and brain sciences and the ways that different configurations of neurological, psychological and physiological theories and their attendant technologies have allowed the self and the world to be rescripted or reimagined in different ways.

The idea of a clash or confusion between different modes of time is often held up as a characteristic of the postmodern age, but this tension between temporalities has long been a feature of the sciences of mind and brain. Since the first emergence of psychological medicine at the beginning of the nineteenth century, we can distinguish at least five different temporalities that have been invoked by practitioners in the field.[1] First, and perhaps most obviously, there is to the lived time of present experience: the time that is captured in simple psychological experiments and reported in a patient's complaints. Such experiences, however, are made meaningful through reference to other temporalities: to the developmental time of individual biography and the evolutionary time in which the organization of our nervous systems was apparently laid out. Alongside these times we can also identify other temporalities: the historical time of changing political, social and cultural values in which scientific claims are made; the future time which is promised in psychological and neuroscientific discoveries or threatened in epidemiological forecasts; the micro-time of intracellular action, the virtual time of computer-based simulations of brain function; and sacred time, beyond conventional or human temporality, which remains a reference point in Western and Eastern religion.

It is the first three of these temporalities – present, developmental and evolutionary time – which for the most part dominate popular understandings of psychology and neuroscience. We see ourselves as creatures with archaic nervous systems, blighted or hamstrung by our childhood experiences and confronting the unprecedented challenges thrown up by modern life. Yet we are also comforted by the promise of a 'neurofuture' or 'cerebral singularity': an eschatological moment in which our carnal limitations will be overcome through advances in the sciences of mind and brain. (Fuller, 2013; Kurzweil, 2009; for a critical view, see Stadler, 2012).

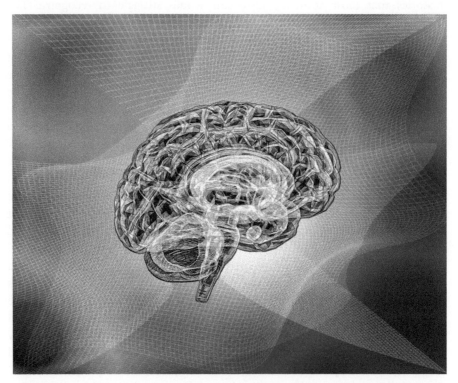

FIGURE 7.1: Model of the human brain. Human Brain Project. Credit: Olga Sabarova / Alamy Stock Photo.

This idea that we stand at an emancipatory moment has been undergirded by significant financial commitments to the neurosciences by western governments. Beginning in July 1989 with George Bush Sr.'s proclamation that the 1990s would be 'the decade of the brain', large scale funding was channelled towards developing new fMRI imaging technologies and encouraging public education and dialogue around the neurosciences. In Europe, the European Commission Seventh Framework Programme invested 1 billion euros in the Human Brain Project – a multi-centre collaborative exercise in which neuroscientists and computer programmers are attempting to build large-scale computer simulation of the working brain. In Japan, India and China, national neuroscientific institutes have been established to continue this work. Built into these contemporary investments and infrastructure, as many commentators have noted, is the promise of physical well-being and cultural change (Moreira and Palladino, 2005). These developments hold out the prospect of a new form of living in which the inner life and the social world are reimagined in biological terms (cf. Abi-Rached and Rose, 2013). They suggest that at some future point, our friendships, habits, desires, political schemes and urban plans could all be benchmarked through reference to the activity of the brain (Fitzgerald et al., 2016).

As some historians have wryly noted, such promises have a long history (Caspar, 2014). Nevertheless, it would probably be a mistake to underestimate the extent to which these governmental investments in the contemporary neurosciences instil a changed relationship to time. Few people stood outside a county lunatic asylum in the nineteenth century and felt the promise of a better future, and the same is probably true for the mental health clinics of the twentieth century. Post-war developments in the neurosciences have brought about a striking reconfiguration in our understanding of transcendence and temporality. Whereas in the Christian West the flesh was for centuries seen as an aspect of our finitude that needed to be overcome through spiritual struggles and inhibition (1 Corinthians 15.21–3, 45–.), the brain and body have now become the pathways to our salvation. The idea of transcendence held out here is peculiar for many reasons. It abandons the old idea of salvation involving an escape from carnal or earthly time (2 Cor. 4:18) to suggest instead that we will be transformed through our identification and engagement with the evolutionary past hardwired into the nervous system. For example, the sociologist Steve Fuller suggests that involvement with the popular literature neuroscience might be enough to transform us into new kind person. As he breathlessly concludes a recent overview of neurohistory: 'focus on the brain encourages our merging with the artifices that enhance our capacity to become attuned to a reality beyond the confines of the biologically given Homo sapiens' (Fuller, 2014: 109; cf. Fuller, 2013: ch. 4). This is a curious kind of spiritual exercise. It is a meditation on the prehistoric time of neurohistory rather than sacred or divine time that brings about our salvation.

NEUROSCIENCE AS A CHALLENGE TO HISTORY

This elevation of prehistoric time in contemporary psychiatry, psychology and popular culture poses a particular challenge for historians (della Rocca, 2015; Cooter, 2014). It promotes the idea that our ordinary desires and everyday responses were somehow scripted outside historical time: in a prehistorical moment that the child psychiatrist, John Bowlby termed the 'Environment of Earliest Adaptation' (EEA) (1969: ch. 4).[2] In the emergent specialism of neurohistory, the champions of this new approach argue that the bringing together of different temporalities – the historical and the prehistoric – can be seen as a vital step in overcoming the parochialism of contemporary history and thus recognizing how our lives are shaped by global, environmental and biological factors (Brooke and Larsen, 2016; Smail and Shyrock, 2013). Thus, in his discussion of the casual aggression of castellans in eleventh- and twelfth-century Europe, Smail argues that their resort to explosive violence was not driven by historical circumstances such as moral collapse or cultural disruption but instead marked the awakening of innate behaviours directed toward the establishment and maintenance of primitive dominance hierarchies. Such hierarchies, he claimed, had all but disappeared in the Paleolithic era when goods were evenly distributed and coalitions of weak individuals would act in consort to suppress rivals that threatened to usurp power (Smail, 2008: 164–70). However, the introduction of agriculture and the production of surplus goods in the Neolithic revolution reintroduced inequality creating an ecology that allowed for the re-emergence of the alpha individual and the reactivation of affective strategies laid down in the nervous system during the EEA. Random violence, according to Smail, 'is just one of the new many new psychotropic mechanisms that evolved to reinstill the feeling of dominance and submission among inferiors in Neo- and Postlithic human societies' (Smail, 2008: 170). It is a routine which anticipates, or implicitly acknowledges, our knowledge of the brain's plasticity. As he notes: '[c]onstant repetition [of violence] could well have induced the formation of specific neural maps or sets of receptors' (2008: 169). The invocation of neural plasticity, prehistoric temporality and the biology of aggression allows for the making of new historical narratives and new historical connections drawing together the micro-histories of local humiliations and economic history of the Mediterranean.

Smail portrays his slippage between medieval scholarship and evolutionary psychiatry as a radical move. He presents his turn to prehistory as an inclusive gesture, one that parallels the recovery of histories of the working classes or colonized peoples that had traditionally been excluded from the historical record. Others have been less convinced. For Roger Cooter, writing in *Isis* in 2014, Smail's approach marked 'a return to a new kind of biological naturalism'. As Cooter went on to explain, 'The body, with the brain now collapsed into it, is re-essentialized, and the act of doing so (which removes human agency from

history, leaving only neural agency) is not acknowledged in itself as ideological'
(2014: 152). The nervous system, fielded in these analyses, is ideological,
Cooter argues, insofar as it incarnates the logic of neoliberalism. It depicts
'human nature as entirely self-interested and incapable of thinking beyond the
market' (2014:153) while foreclosing the possibility of change. Such models
ignore the contingency of our current understandings of the brain and mind (cf.
Cooter 2013: 165). Certainly an easy parallel can be drawn between the
contemporary injunction in liberal societies towards self-improvement and self-
care and the widespread acceptance of neuroplasticity with its idea that the
brain can be transformed through personal effort and training (Pitts-Taylor,
2010). At the same time, it is also clear that this approach is contingent.
Alternative neurological theories have sustained very different visions of human
history. In the early 1970s, Michael Gazzaniga's and Roger Sperry's work on
the lateralization of brain function was used to underwrite the historical claims
made in Julian Jaynes' *The Origins of Consciousness in the Breakdown of the
Bicameral Mind* (1976). Our sense of personal agency and self-consciousness,
were, Jaynes argued, quite recent historical phenomena that had emerged
around 2,000 years ago, some time between the writing of the *Iliad* and the
Odyssey.

Smail and Jaynes present dramatic examples of the ways that particular
understandings of the nervous system make different kinds of historical
narrative possible. Although superficially eccentric, they should also stand to
make us aware of the implicit understandings of brain, mind and agency that
inform all historical narratives. Sometimes these understandings are contested,
as in the ongoing disputes over the history of emotions, but most of the time
they are ignored. There is no approach to history that can escape the problems
of neurological or psychological reflexivity (Smith, 2005). And there is of
course, no understanding of brain and mind that can escape ideology, although
the ideological work produced through the broad approaches of the
neurosciences is open ended and always susceptible to re-appropriation. Thus,
the evolutionary psychologies that underpin the neurohistories of Smail and his
colleagues are often seen as a rehash of the right-wing sociobiological theories
that circulated in the 1970s (Segerstråle, 2000). While they do share a common
structure and reference points, it is also clear that such theories can provide the
grounds for very different forms of political action. It is a commonplace
nowadays to hear left-wing commentators complain that under neoliberalism
'human beings, the ultrasocial mammals, whose brains are wired to respond to
other people, are being peeled apart' (Monbiot, 2013) or that social inequality
triggers primitive forms of depressive reaction (James, 2008; Fisher, 2009:
ch. 3). Drawing together different temporalities – the primitive and the present
– through reference to the objects of modern neuroscience provides the
foundation for contemporary critique.

MAKING TEMPORALITIES IN THE MODERN SCIENCES OF MIND AND BRAIN

Although the neurosciences might provide the foundational temporalities for current political critiques, they do not provide a steady foundation. Even the most cursory survey of the history of the mind and brain sciences reveals how very different understandings and experiences of time have emerged as various complexes of techniques, classifications, objectives and institutions coalesced at different moments around different problems. Psychological medicine as a distinct form of practice emerged at the beginning of the nineteenth century around the administrative problems of criminal insanity and safeguarding the insane. Yet even within the first hundred years of its existence, its bases, goals and techniques would be transformed and a very different form of temporality would be produced in asylum work.

The first therapeutic asylums, as opposed to custodial madhouses or religious sanctuaries, had been established in the closing decades of the eighteenth century. Pioneer alienists, including Philippe Pinel in Paris, Vincenzo Chiarugi in Tuscany, Benjamin Rush in Philadelphia and William Tuke in York saw the asylum as a therapeutic instrument that would operate upon the disordered ideas of a deranged mind by imposing a new sensory regime. Working with the sensationalist philosophy of John Locke, they organised the asylum as a bricks and mortar machine that would subject the patient to a constant flow of reassuring and respectable experiences that would encourage the construction of new ideas and associations in the suffering patient (Gauchet and Swain, 1999). Tuke and Pinel arranged the asylum as a kind of therapeutic theatre in which various ruses and subterfuges (concealed bars, muffled locks) disguised from the patient the reality of their condition, while at the same time bourgeois entertainments (tea parties, Arcadian vistas, prayer meetings, rabbits and domesticated seagulls) were used to encourage the return to health (Tuke, 1814/1996: 96).

Although this approach (termed 'the moral treatment' by its advocates) is often seen as an anticipation of contemporary psychotherapeutic treatment because of its prioritization of the psychological over the physical and its emphasis on the restorative power of personal relationships, this comparison rests upon a misapprehension. In contrast to contemporary therapy, the alienists were not interested in the patient's past. Instead, as we have just seen, they saw illness in architectonic terms: as a form of derangement that could be overcome by the reordering of ideas and sensations. Medicine's turn to the patient's developmental past and later, their evolutionary past, was in large part driven by the early failures of the asylum. By the middle decades of the nineteenth century, it was clear that many patients were not being rescued by the asylum. Instead the institutions were silting up long-stay inmates, a growth in numbers that made it difficult to recreate the atmosphere of bourgeois domesticity that had been foundational to the moral treatment.

This therapeutic failure, and the accumulation of long stay patients in the institution, had a number of effects. At one level, as a generation of psychiatric historians have noted, it led to a crisis of professional confidence among alienists who sought forms of legitimacy for their institutions now that the asylum had lost its therapeutic rationale (Scull, 1993). At another level, the organization of asylums opened up a new perspective on illness. The institution presented its inmates as a distinct population whose symptoms and behaviour could be observed across the life course and whose pathological histories could be compared to those of their fellow patients and to normal lives achieved by citizens of the outside world. It was a 'museum of madness', which displayed the psychopathologies of its patients across developmental and evolutionary time.

By the beginning of the twentieth century, the asylum was operating as a machine that produced a very particular kind of knowledge – case histories in which the subject's physique and behaviour could be tracked and compared through index files and folders and eventually correlated with post-mortem reports (Weber and Engstrom, 2007). This interest in tracking the temporal unfolding of disease – and the inability to observe patients once they had been discharged from the asylum – led to a shift in classification. There was a growing faith in the existence of stable entities rather than transformative experiences that organized the shape and progress of mental disease. Deep interest in the aetiology of 'general paresis of the insane' – an illness which progressed from psychological symptoms to spinal paralysis – stabilized around the idea of syphilitic infection in the 1890s. At the same time, Emil Kraepelin, the director of the Psychiatric Clinic at the University of Heidelberg, exploited the clinic's rich records to demonstrate that progressive degeneration in many patients followed a distinct pattern. In the fourth edition of his *Textbook on Psychiatry* (1893), he argued that this progressive illness, 'dementia praecox', and an oscillating affective illness (cyclothymia – which he would later term manic depressive insanity) formed the twin bases of the endogenous mental illnesses (Engstrom, 2003). It was the asylum's custodial function and its administrative machinery that rendered these illnesses visible.

This brief sketch shows how a mixture of economic pressures, judicial decisions and welfare reforms could work together through the asylum to open up a developmental or biographical perspective on mental illness. It was the combination of this new perspective, with the professionalizing turn to pathological anatomy and asylum laboratory research, that would in turn provide some stability for the working classifications of illness developed by the early alienists. The turn to cerebral anatomy and the comparison of developing and declining brains would help to introduce an evolutionary perspective on to the sufferings of the brain injured and the insane.

From the middle decades of the nineteenth century, there was an ongoing attempt to map functional loss onto lesions in the brain. The work of Paul

Broca and colleagues in France on the localization of aphasia held out the hope that changes in capacity and personality could be reliably traced in the failures of the flesh. At the same time, the growing literature in the physiological psychology of Marshall Hall and Wilhelm Griesinger on reflex activity in the brain and spinal cord paved the way for an evolutionary understanding of mental illness as the surrender of consciousness to automatism (Jacyna, 2000). This definition, which dovetailed neatly with legal ideas around forensic responsibility, was developed by the English neurologist Hughlings Jackson. He depicted mental disease as an atavistic process involving the dissolution of the higher nervous centres. Drawing upon his studies of epilepsy at the National Hospital, Queen Square, Jackson argued that seizures represented a process of disinhibition in which lower more primitive processes were suddenly given free rein (Smith, 1992: 162–7).

Although it was often difficult to demonstrate at post mortem the processes that Jackson had imagined, the brains of syphilitics and those diagnosed with general paresis of the insane provided telling examples of the brain's decay. The 'softened' tissue of the syphilitic's brain, which often collapsed during dissection, demanded the discovery of new histological and surgical techniques (such as the invention of the microtome in 1875 and the use of tissue stains) as well as new recording methods, photography, resin brain casts and printed diagrams for logging the distribution of lesions (Wallis, 2017: ch. 3; Hakosalo, 2006). The discovery of astrocytes or 'spider cells' conglomerating in the brains of syphilitics provided a dramatic example of how the brain's regression into atavistic disorganization could be made visible by the new anatomical techniques of the late nineteenth century. Through the use of tissues stains and microtomes the working judgements of nineteenth-century alienists were now anchored in evolutionary time.

MANAGING THE PAST IN MODERN PSYCHOLOGICAL MEDICINE

The discovery of these new temporalities – the evolutionary time of atavistic brain and the lived time of the unconscious nervous system – opened up a new vista of work for the discipline of psychological medicine. Members of the nascent psychiatric profession began to frame their purpose in eugenic terms, recognizing that although the asylum could not save the individual, it could still safeguard the future of the race. The profession's task now lay in the management of history and sexuality: challenges it pursued through two superficially different yet intimately connected scientific projects, psychoanalysis and psychiatric genetics. These two projects are now generally seen as representing distinct traditions, but both arose from a common commitment to the management of history (encoded in either personal memory or biological inheritance) and sexuality, which from the end of the nineteenth century was understood as a complex of instincts specific to each individual that had been scripted in a primitive past. The attempt to manage the life of populations, which Foucault termed biopolitics, was borne from the opening up of these new forms of temporality in the brain and mind sciences (Foucault, 2003; for suggestive remarks, see Berlant, 2007).

The eugenic approach drew upon the development of new psychometric instruments. Alfred Binet's test of individual psychology (1895) and Charles Spearman's test of general intelligence (1904) allowed for the measure of individual capacity and its distribution across the population. With the contemporaneous rise of compulsory education and personnel selection in the military, the tests provided a means for identifying defective individuals within a population and for comparing the relative capacities of different populations. Failing individuals and colonized peoples could be understood as throwbacks to an earlier age. Nineteenth-century concerns with idiots and incurables were reframed in terms of the threat to the evolutionary present. The biopolitical programmes that arose from this approach are well known. As historians have shown, they legitimated a range of interventions from the establishment of epileptic colonies and maternal welfare programmes through to the mass sterilization and extermination enacted under the Nazis' Aktion T4 regime.

The turn to eugenics and psychoanalysis was driven by a Darwinian understanding of the psyche, which depicted selfhood as a fragile achievement built upon an unruly repertoire of inherited responses. Yet it was also promoted by a conspicuous shift in the presentation of illness. In the closing decades of the nineteenth century, there was a startling growth in hysteria: an illness that appeared to have been shaped in opposition to European and North American definitions of sanity. The Victorian asylum system, caught up as it was in processes of legal and political administration, drew an equivalence between psychological health and the achievement of personal agency and responsibility. It was an equivalence that was reinforced in nineteenth-century psychophysiology which pathologized automatism as an example of nervous atavism. Hysteria turned these professional judgements into a public language. The fits, paralyses and fainting episodes that became a characteristic of *fin-de-siècle* life were a dramatic representation of the failure of personal agency. It was in this context that memory became the zone of medical intervention.

In the wards supervised by Jean-Martin Charcot at the Salpêtrière Hospital in Paris, patients' bodies traced out the divisions and limitations of their personalities demonstrating fugues, amnesias, paralyses, aphasias, visual disturbances and anaesthesias. Charcot suggested that these psychic injuries were a product of hereditary weakness with the personality splintering and fragmenting in response to shock and trauma. In this account, the subconscious was a temporary artefact, produced through experiences of extreme stress, and could be reintegrated through hypnotic intervention. In the hands of Charcot's colleagues and rivals, Frederic Myers and Pierre Janet, this therapeutic task became more complex. It was a literary endeavour, in which therapist and patient sought to achieve a coherent plot out of present behaviour and a recovered past, and it opened up a new market for self-work outside the asylum as private practitioners embraced the possibility of office psychiatry. The subconscious developmental past, lost through trauma or weakness, became the objects of psychotherapy. Recovery, as Janet insisted, lay in a process of 'presentification' in which temporal order would be re-established. As Janet explained towards the end of his career, the patient must be able to 'associate a happening with the other events of his life, how to put it in its place in that life history which for each of us is an essential element in personality' (Janet, 1925: 662).

The significance of Sigmund Freud's project – and that of his followers in the psychoanalytic movement – lay in his integration of this remedial work on the recovery of developmental time with the evolutionary or animal time of sexuality. Initially Freud shared the literary approach to hysterical symptoms, but soon departed from Myers and Janet in his insistence that the disruptive power of traumatic memories stemmed from their connection to the sexual instincts. Having initially insisted that these sexual traumas originated in episodes of childhood seduction and abuse, by the early years of the twentieth century he was arguing that this process of repression was universal, being triggered by the incestuous fantasies that were an inevitable (albeit socially unacceptable) aspect of modern childhood. The genius of the psychoanalytic position, with its insistence on the universality of what Freud termed the Oedipus complex, was that it made everyone the potential subject of therapeutic intervention.

We can discern a twofold process taking place in Freud's arguments. First, the unconscious was transformed from being a temporary artefact produced through traumatic episodes to become an enduring aspect of the personality. At the same time, the hysterical condition was universalized, rendering every individual the subject of psychiatric or psychological expertise. Grounding these rhetorical claims rested upon the achievement of new alliances with experimental psychology and electrophysiology. The appearance of new technologies in the middle decades of the nineteenth century, such as the kymograph (a simple stylus on a mercury float that continuously recorded on a clockwork powered rotating drum) allowed constant recordings to be made of physiological changes such as pulse or blood pressure (de Chadarevian, 1993). In combination with tools such as the manometer and the galvanometer, accurate readings of physiological changes in bodily capacities such as blood pressure or skin conductivity were recorded and read as signs of emotional arousal. The discrepancy between verbally reported feelings and the changes revealed by the instrument provided a telling demonstration of the existence of bodily time: internal processes unfolding to very different rhythms and responding to stimuli outside conscious experience (Borck, 2016; Dror, 2001).

PLASTICITY, THE ADAPTIVE PSYCHE AND THE DISCOVERY OF THE PSYCHOSOCIAL WORLD

The insurance machinery of the early welfare states, like the asylum earlier, made visible the evolutionary and developmental temporalities of their populations. Local and national differences in educational achievement, patterns of reproduction and asylum admission rates served as ready indices of biological difference across the population. However, whereas these prototypical indicators simply revealed a landscape of biological difference with different social and economic arrangements sustaining pockets of poor inheritance or evolutionary progress, in the twentieth century a much more complex relationship between society and psychological temporality emerged. This new perspective was sustained, in part, by a growing interest in the adaptive capacities of the human brain: an interest that was deepened and reinforced by the psychiatric catastrophe of the First World War.

The interest in the brain's adaptive capacities was in part inspired by Jackson's evolutionary neurology, but in the hands of his most influential follower, Charles Scott Sherrington, there was a much greater emphasis on the achievement of individuality in an unstable environment. In *The Integrative Action of the Nervous System* (1906), Sherrington outlined how man's higher nature and purpose was won though the successful combination of individual reflex actions. Through this action, Sherrington argued, 'the nervous system unifies from separate organs an animal possessing solidarity, an individual' (Sherrington, 1906: 2; Smith, 2003). The human mind and brain were no longer the fixed objects, imagined by eugenicists and localizationists: they possessed a dynamic capacity to respond and adapt to the challenges laid down by the environment.

This modernist faith in the dynamic and adaptive capacities of the mind and brain found clear expression during the psychiatric emergency of the First World War. From a neurological perspective, the war could be regarded as a 'physio-pathological experiment on a grand scale' (Pieron, 1927: 4). The thousands of head injuries sustained in conflict encouraged a new suspicion of what the existentialist psychiatrist, Karl Jaspers would later call 'brain mythologies': the idea of an easy match between functional loss and neurological damage. A new generation of holistic neurologists including Kurt Goldstein and Karl Lashley followed Sherrington in arguing that purposive action was coordinated across the whole cerebral cortex. From this viewpoint, the patterns of functional loss exhibited in brain injuries were not simple static reflections of local damage but fluid reports of the patient's pattern of recovery (Geroulanos and Meyers, 2016).

This pattern of recovery could itself be pathological. For the American physiologists Walter Cannon and George Crile, it was the body's response to insult and injuries that also threatened to destroy it. Crile and Cannon brought together ideas of evolutionary temporality and present response, arguing that the body responded to environmental challenges through the activation of the primitive systems of the endocrine glands and the autonomic nervous system. Prolonged activation of these systems generated a series of pathological effects ranging from gastric ulcers through to leucocytosis. These responses were pathological because they were out of step with modern time. As Crile explained, 'man has reached his present status of civilization with brutish organs . . . And now, though sitting at this desk in command of the complicated machinery of civilization, when he fears a business catastrophe his fear is manifested in the terms of his ancestral physical battle in the struggle for existence' (Crile, 1915: 61–2; Hayward, 2013: 232–3).

These theories of neural plasticity and adaptive response served to undermine the idea that mental illness could be seen in terms of evolutionary regression or hereditary weakness. It was no longer the simple destiny of the unfit but a complex reaction to the challenges of modern life. Illness was now seen in psychosocial terms, a perspective reinforced by the mass outbreaks of nervous disorder thrown up in the conflict. The shared psychological suffering of officers and rank and file democratized mental illness encouraging the idea that the fault lay outside the flesh in the perverse ecology of war (Barham, 2004). Illness was now seen as an unhappy accident, generated by the challenges of life, a view that found its clearest expression the 'psychobiology' of the Swiss American, Adolf Meyer. Meyerian psychobiology, although garlanded with an extremely technical vocabulary of 'parergasias' and 'merergasic reactions', encouraged a common-sense approach in which the patient's life course was charted for stressful life events that could evoke the pattern of breakdown (Leys, 1991).

At the same time that the link with ancestral inheritance was thus weakened, the signs of stress were vastly multiplied. The idea of pathological response allowed many different forms of illness to be read as symptoms of environmental mismatch. Franz Alexander, a pioneer of the new school of psychosomatic medicine identified what he called the 'magic seven' symptoms: bronchial asthma, essential hypertension, rheumatoid arthritis, peptic ulceration, ulcerative colitis, hyperthyroidism and neurodermatitis. His colleagues, such as Helen Flanders Dunbar and James Halliday, vastly expanded the list. The sick body could now be read as a kind of carnal commentary on the psychological costs of modern living. The vast number of sickness cases recorded in the administrative machinery of the welfare states also allowed this temporal disjuncture to be read on a national scale. The apparatus of national insurance and workmen's compensation opened up a new epidemiological perspective on mental health. It shifted from a focus on those legally judged to be insane to become something that was problematized across the population. Social policies and state planning now became the instruments of individual mental health. In the work of groups such as the Chicago School sociologists and the Rockefeller Foundation Committee on the Relationships of Sociology and Psychiatry, the social environment was reimagined as a landscape of psychiatric risk.

The relationship between individual and environment now began to be understood in new terms. Whereas in the early studies of adaptation and in psychoanalysis the environment had been seen as frustrating primitive instincts and authentic desires, by the 1930s a number of renegade psychoanalysts, including Wilhelm Stekel, Trigant Burrow and Ian Suttie, began to argue that subjectivity was rooted in social life. Their position was reinforced by studies published by the Culture and Personality school of anthropologists, most notably Margaret Mead's studies of sexuality in Western Samoa, which demonstrated how the most intimate aspects of the interior life were bound up with patterns of social organization (Levine, 2001). The psyche was seen as a social achievement, and its pathologies, as Karen Horney insisted, were brought about by the capitalist promotion of competitive autonomy that frustrated the innate biological need to love (Horney, 1937).

During the Second World War, the belief that social security and community cohesion would serve as a prophylaxis against mental breakdown became central to public policy. In the United Kingdom, systems of national surveillance were instituted to safeguard the blitzed population against neurotic breakdown. At the end of the war, new international organizations, such as the World Federation of Mental Health and the World Health Organization, promoted the idea that internal and external stability could only be achieved through the pursuit of social experiments in mental hygiene. Experiments in which the individual was encouraged to exercise personal autonomy while at the same time recognizing their rootedness in the family and community (Toms, 2013). Psychiatrists experimented with ward organization, operating limited forms of open-door policy while attempting to coordinate with local authorities and national charities to extend the care and surveillance into community care.

ELECTROPHYSIOLOGY AND THE DISSOLUTION OF THE ADAPTIVE PSYCHE

From the 1920s through to the 1950s, there was an ongoing attempt to harness the adaptive potential of the nervous system to bring about a process of recalibration in the mentally ill. Convulsive treatments such as insulin coma therapy, cardiazol shock and electro-convulsive therapy were all developed during the 1920s and 1930s, with the intention of triggering a process that would shock the nervous system back into a state of homeostasis. Similarly the deployment of surgical therapies such as leucotomy (developed by Egas Moniz, a Portuguese surgeon and politician, in 1935) held out hope that deliberate damage would induce a process of self-correction. In attempting to harness the dynamic properties of the brain, these therapies helped to popularize the idea that there was no authentic self to be recovered, just the possibility that a more effective balance could be achieved.

Increasingly, operation of the nervous system, and the individual personality, were both seen in a kind of equivalence with the tools and technologies that had been developed to investigate them. The development of new forms of electrophysiological investigation, particularly the electroencephalograph (EEG) pioneered by Hans Berger in 1936 and popularized by W. G. Lennox in the US and William Grey Walter in the UK, promoted the idea that 'electricity was the

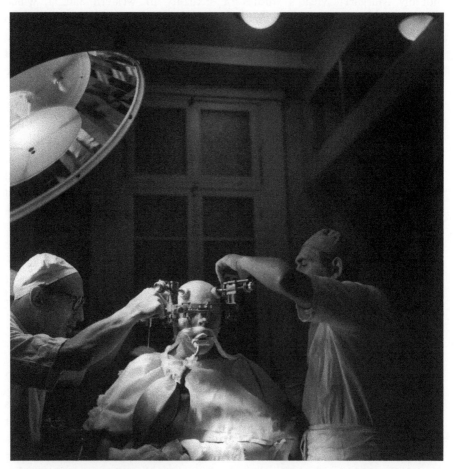

FIGURE 7.2: Psychosurgery with a stereoaxic device, Paris, Saint-Anne Hospital, 1954. Credit: Jean-Phillipe CHARBONNIER / Contributor / Getty Images.

medium of psychic life' and that the long sought after authentic interior would simply be a transient pattern within broader flows of electrical information (Borck, 2001). With the growth of cybernetic science in the late 1940s, a broad coalition of mathematicians, psychiatrists, anthropologists and engineers argued that problems of mind and behaviour could be reconceptualized in terms of the flow of information. Automata, such as the homeostat and the mechanical tortoise, were constructed to model the self-correcting powers of the adaptive psyche and demonstrate the ways that complex behaviour could be produced through the combination and integration of simple reflex actions. It was a mechanical model of the psyche that elided the ancestral past, in favour of a new focus upon present response.

Similarly psychiatrists now began to view mental pathology as stemming from the disruption of flows of information. At the Langley Porter Neuropsychiatric Institute in California, the psychiatrist Jurgen Ruesch, working with the anthropologist Gregory Bateson, argued that psychosomatic illness among recent immigrants could be attributed to failures of communication. Blocked signals would leak out as behavioural disturbances or physical symptoms. Likewise at the Maudsley Hospital in London, George Brown and his colleagues were able to refigure the onset of schizophrenia as a response to frustrations in domestic communication. This cybernetic reading of schizophrenia as an adaptive response to familial frustration received its clearest exegesis in the work of the radical psychiatrist R. D. Laing. Laing combined Bateson's theory of the double-bind with the existential analysis of personal identity developed by Jean-Paul Sartre to develop a theory of mental illness as a strategic response to the challenge of distorted communication (Laing, 1961).

We can see how Bateson and Laing's insights into the pathological costs of disordered communication flattened out the historical temporality that had been built up in early twentieth-century psychiatry and psychoanalysis. Illness was not the outcome of an inherited condition or a frustrated ancestral biology; rather, it stemmed from present tensions. Although most psychiatrists never fully embraced the reduction of illness to distorted communication, the cybernetic programme encouraged an ecological turn in psychiatry, as practitioners sought to map out the implication of patterns of social organization, whether in the ward or the patient's family, upon mental health. The parallel growth of clinical psychology encouraged the development of pragmatic forms of psychotherapy – the behavioural and cognitive behavioural therapies – that eschewed the search for authenticity in favour of strategies for behaviour modification.

The growth of these new behavioural therapies was tied up with the development of psychiatric rating scales which had developed out of wartime selection procedures to provide a standardized method for screening psychiatric admissions and for a case-finding in the wider community. Paper instruments such as the Minnesota Multiphasic Personality Inventory (first developed in

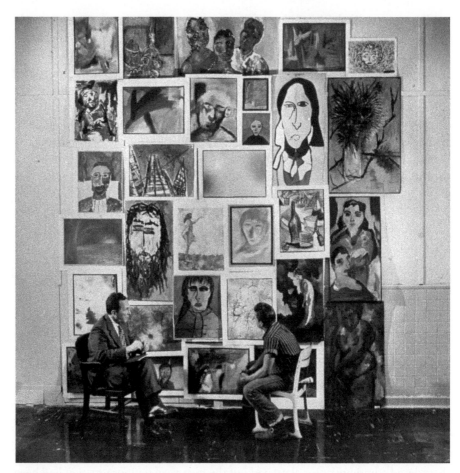

FIGURE 7.3: Psychiatrist with an emotionally disturbed student, in front of paintings by emotionally disturbed students at special school. Credit: Fritz Goro / Contributor / Getty.

1940 and refined in 1952), the Maudsley Personality Inventory (1959) and Max Hamilton's rating scales for anxiety (1959) and depression (1960) promoted the idea that illness was not a discrete entity but instead a form of behaviour which existed upon a spectrum from normality to abnormality. From this perspective, the task of therapy was readjustment of behaviour.

The first wave of behavioural therapies, inspired by the theories of Ivan Pavlov and J. B. Watson, trained patients to address phobias and sexual perversions through a process of reward ('operant conditioning') or overexposure ('systematic desensitization') (Browne, 1967). By 1970, this simple focus on behaviour modification had been expanded to include strategies on managing interior thought and in particular the interpretation of events and experience. The rise of rational emotive behaviour therapy and cognitive behavioural therapy pioneered by Albert Ellis and Aaron Beck, respectively, in the late 1960s worked to blur the boundary between clinical psychology and popular and growing post-war literature on self-improvement. The mind was now increasingly seen as a project which would repay considerable investment. Indeed in the hands of humanistic psychologists, such as Carl Rogers and Albert Maslow, therapy became the first step in a process of forward projection that would allow for the unleashing of human potential (Maslow, 1970 [1964]). The ease with which such interventions could be enacted, however, raised new concerns over the vulnerability of the subject. These concerns found clear expression in the literature on brainwashing: a subject that neatly drew together post-war fears around the overwhelming effects of new media such as film with ethical concerns around the power of psychiatry and psychiatrists. (Holmes, 2017; Killen and Andriopoulos, 2011).

PSYCHOPHARMACOLOGY AND THE RETURN OF HISTORY

The paper instruments deployed in post-war psychiatric assessment and cognitive behavioural therapies had the effect of flattening out time. They collapsed past and future into the present situation. They aimed to capture the patient's condition, locate it upon a spectrum of responses and suggest strategies for overcoming the situation – either through mental exercises or through simple pharmaceutical interventions. The 1950s and 1960s had witnessed a dramatic expansion in the psychopharmacological armamentarium as treatment regimes moved beyond the asylum into the wider community. Following the commercial success of the antipsychotic chlorpromazine (largactil) from 1952, there was intense investment in psychopharmacological experimentation leading to the emergence of a new range of now-familiar minor tranquillizers (meprobamate/Miltown (1955)), benzodiazepines (Librium (1960) and Valium (1963)) and anti-depressants (imipramine (1957) and amitryptiline (1961)).

The rapid growth of pharmacotherapy and the related rating instruments had a number of effects. On the one hand, as Sonu Shamdasani and Mikkel Borch Jacobsen has argued, they served as vehicles for a particular neurochemical version of human nature, encouraging patients to interrogate their feelings in particular ways and assess their findings against a norm abstracted from the broader community (Borch-Jacobsen, 2009). On the other, as Andrew Scull and others have claimed, the fact that psychiatric judgements and treatment decisions were now based on self-reports and consensual agreement left the psychiatric enterprise wide open to critique (Scull, 2015: 378–402). It was simply a form of game playing in which patients and physicians either struggled for authority or conspired together to define themselves in mutually beneficial roles

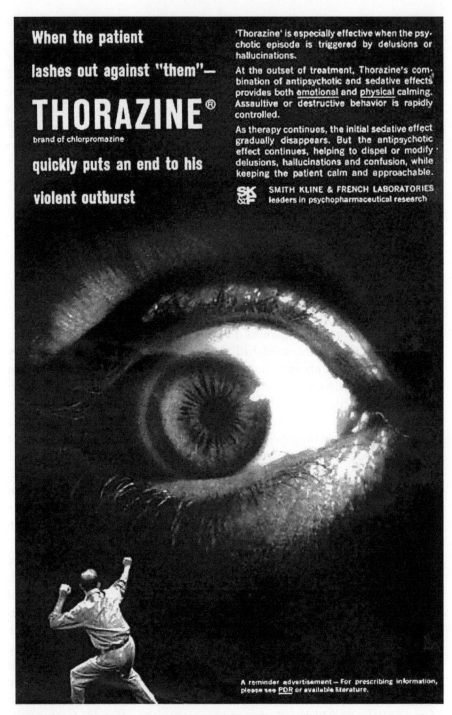

FIGURE 7.4: Thorazine advertisement, Smith, Klein, and French Laboratories, circa 1960. Credit: Archive PL / Alamy Stock Photo.

(Szasz, 1961/1973). The fact that health, in the post-war period, was increasingly seen in terms of successful social adjustment only reinforced the sense that psychiatry was simply becoming another tool for achieving political consensus.

The growth of countercultural critiques during the 1950s and internal attacks such as the Rosenhan experiment (in which healthy students were admitted to mental hospitals after simply reporting at interview that they repeatedly heard the words 'thud' or 'empty'), led to a new attempt to establish the bases of psychiatric work. This was pursued in part through an attempt to formalize psychiatric diagnosis and standardize judgements (Casey, 2017). Robert Spitzer and colleagues led a task force to overhaul the third edition of the Diagnostic and Statistical Manual (DSM) of the American Psychiatric Association arguing for the introduction of strict tests of statistical validity, drawn from the criteria developed by John Feighner to demonstrate the stability of diagnostic categories over time. Although the Research Diagnostic Criteria established by Spitzer and colleagues overthrew much of the psychoanalytic inheritance that had shaped working definitions in US psychiatry, they remained detached from contemporary work in biology. This detachment was surprising given the wealth of data that was emerging from developments in neuro-imaging and claims to biological specificity made by new generation of anti-depressants, the Selective Serotonin Reuptake Inhibitors (SSRIs) that appeared on the market at this time.

The rebiologization of psychological medicine and the mind sciences that took place during the 1980s brought with it a reassertion of evolutionary temporality. Drawing upon the affect theories developed by Silvan Tomkins and his followers in the 1960s, illnesses were again seen as forms of primitive response hardwired into the circuitry of the human brain. Social factors that had dominated in interwar theories were now reduced to biological triggers, provoking set routines that had been scripted in the prehistoric past. Thus in the work of John Price, depression was interpreted as an adaptive response. It was mechanism for encouraging weak and defeated animals to withdraw from the group, reducing the recurrence of infighting and encouraging the social cohesion and individual survival (Young, 2001). Pharmacology allowed these scripted processes to be disrupted, holding out the prospect that our evolutionary past could be engaged with through pharmaceutical means. At the same time, this past was held up as a stable ground for psychiatric classification, as researchers searched for the specific neurological affect programmes that underlay individual disorders. As the Director of the US National Institute of Mental Health, explained in justification of the Institute's decision to abandon the DSM: 'It has become our mantra at NIMH that disorders can be addressed as disorders of the brain circuits' (quoted in Casey, 2017: 229). Evolutionary temporality had now returned as the grounds of truth.

HISTORY, NEUROSCIENCE AND THE ENGINE OF TEMPORALITIES

Throughout the twentieth century, the mind and brain have served as the meeting point for different temporalities: temporalities that have been made visible and articulated through different and various techniques, technologies, theories, institutions and policies. It is also clear that despite the vocal concerns of critics, this constant shifting of temporalities made possible by the mind sciences has not led to the exclusion of historicity or the triumph of essentialism. For philosophers and historians such as Roger Smith and Ian Hacking, the shifts in the way we see ourselves transform human nature (Smith, 2006; Hacking, 2002). The concepts, categories and technologies that we bring to bear on our subjectivity provide the materials through which we live and experience our lives. And as critical neuroscience is now making apparent, these materials go beyond language and culture to include the tools and products of our current labour.

This sense of the determinative role of history and the close involvement of the self, the brain and world has long had enjoyed a following in the mind sciences. In the 1950s, the psychoanalyst Allen Wheelis noted how the patients he encountered in his day-to-day practice in California were very different from

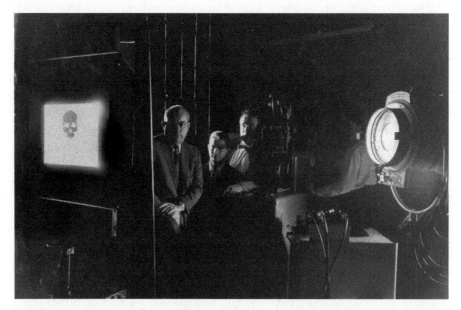

FIGURE 7.5: Movie producer William S. Edwards (L) standing with neurologist Hal C. Becker (C), and psychologist Robert E. Corrigan working on subliminal perception experiments for TV. Credit: Bill Bridges / Contributor / Getty Images.

patients analysed by Freud. They had become a new kind of person. Such a transformation, his contemporary Julian Huxley argued, could be attributed to the work of tools and cultures: instruments that extended the nervous system allowing for the achievement of new capacities (Huxley, 1957; Bashford, 2013). By the 1960s, this idea of culture and technology as prostheses or the extension of man was commonplace in the science of cybernetics, popular literature and media theory (Wolfe, 1953; Young, 1950). By the end of the twentieth century, the sense that we live in an 'age of entanglement' has become central to critical neuroscience. Neuroscience no longer removes us from history; it instead demonstrates how we are made, in part, through the products of lived labour.

Part of the work of historians has been to break down the separation of temporalities to demonstrate that there is no aspect of carnal time that remains insulation from the conditions of its historical production. The turn to evolutionary temporality alarms historians, as it suggests that the wellsprings of human action lie outside language, culture and society. Yet in the work of contemporary neuroscientists such as Andy Clark and Alva Noë, there is a new emphasis on consciousness as a form of practice: a practice which is made possible by the nervous system's involvement with the world. Such accounts allow us to take the role of history in the formation of identity much more seriously. The accumulation of materials, categories, languages, relationships, tools and traditions provides the grounds for identity and action. As Smail himself notes:

> We have incorporated things into our being in much the same way that our distant eukaryotic ancestors incorporated mitochondria and our genome has absorbed autonomous strands of viral DNA. We have always been post/human cyborgs. . . . This quality of plasticity is especially characteristic of the brain. Tools and hammers, for example, literally grow into the map of the body when they are used. They become a curious sort of limb, a prosthesis that can be taken off and put on at will.

> —2014: 115

From this perspective, the mind is not something prescripted in our evolutionary history; rather it is something that is being constantly remade anew under the particular material and economic conditions of the present time. As Marx argued in *Grundrisse*: 'Production thus not only creates an object for the subject, but also a subject for the object' (1857: pt. 1, sect, 2), and we can perhaps extend this analysis to the making of the brain and the making of time. As this chapter has shown, those temporalities which threaten to divide common discourse and support new forms of authority and expertise are themselves contingent productions of the history of the mind and brain sciences.

NOTES

1. This arguments builds upon and extends Pettit and Hegarty's analysis of the interplay of multiple temporalities in the history of sexuality (Pettit and Hegarty, 2013).
2. I recognize that contemporary evolutionary psychologists, following the work of John Tooby and Led Cosmides, argue that EEA does not refer to a defined place or time but rather is a statistical abstraction of the different selection pressures that led to the evolution of a particular adaptation.

CHAPTER EIGHT

Authority

GEORGE WEISZ

'Medical authority' is an ambiguous term. There are two problems with it (as Bruno Latour said about network analysis): the word 'medical' and the word 'authority'. What exactly does medical refer to? The individual physician? The organized medical profession as a whole? Influential professional elites? Definitions of the human conditions? And what about 'authority'? How exactly does it differ from other terms used by social scientists that that cover similar terrain like 'dominance' or 'sovereignty', or even 'power'? And what exactly is the object of this power? Given these limitations, and with the help of several dictionaries, one can come up with the following partial list of features that usually cover the term 'medical authority'.

1. Authority over patients and their actions.
2. Authority to manage the activity of other health professionals.
3. Authority to define the material conditions and organizational structure of health care and its institutions.
4. Authority to define what *is* a disease or disability (which can lead to entitlements) and what is and is not appropriate therapy.
5. And perhaps most common in the scholarly literature, authority to define who is allowed to practice what procedures and what constitute proper standards of training, practice and professional behaviour.

Although each of these meanings of 'medical authority' has a somewhat different historical trajectory, and varies from country to country, there seems to be a general scholarly consensus that medical authority (or dominance or sovereignty), especially over patients, increased during the first half of the twentieth century and that it has been declining since the 1960s and 1970s.[1]

More recent research speaks less about reduction than about the significant transformation of medical authority. This seems a more plausible approach. There is now a body of historical literature that questions whether there was ever a 'golden age' of medical authority. Reviewing several recent books, David Jones argues, 'medical authority has been consistently challenged ever since it first took its modern form in the late nineteenth century. Patients as consumers have repeatedly asserted their right and ability to evaluate critically physicians' claims and to make their own decisions' (Jones, 2017; Engelmann, 2017). By the same token, numerous works in sociology, political science and organizational studies have moved away from the simple notion that there has been a zero-sum transition away from the authority of physicians to that of administrators or patient/consumers. Chamberlain argues that 'instead of being in decline medicine is undergoing a process of restratification whereby the profession increasingly splits into elite and rank and file segments and the former subject the latter to new and more intrusive forms of peer surveillance and control in order to maintain regulatory privileges (albeit in a more publicly accountable form)' (Chamberlain, 2012: vi). Others suggest that like other professions, medicine is now based on more diffuse and hybrid forms of authority that are entirely novel; these may include input from various health care occupations, politicians, administrators, scholars in such fields as health services research, patient and advocacy groups, and techniques for producing metrics and/or consensus decisions (Noordegraaf, 2015). In a study of medical training in the UK and the Netherlands, it is argued, 'professional self-governance has turned into more hybrid forms of coregulation in which the medical profession, the state, and other private actors continuously reinstate their positions and related claims to authority' (Wallenburg et al., 2012: 441). Given the multiple aspects of medical authority, it may well be that different interpretations actually apply to different types of authority.

For the purposes of this chapter, I would like to focus on the self-regulation of physicians, today one of a number of health professions that, so we are told, work together in collaborative fashion, but who nonetheless retain special status. Physician self-regulation has been the source of much discussion for the past half-century and seems somehow near the epicentre of professional physician identity. But as interesting and consequential as social scientists find the balance of power and authority among professional elites, organizational or state authorities, patients and, as we now like to say, 'stakeholders', I propose that another sort of transformation has contributed to changing notions of medical authority. For physicians, such authority is no longer based exclusively on formal professional credentials but increasingly on new techniques of regulation that aim to standardize and improve both physicians and their practices. While the goals of continuing improvement are real enough and are certainly consequential, these techniques also have symbolic value, carrying a reassuring message to the lay world that medical authority guarantees both the safe practice and humanitarian values of physicians.

SOME BASIC CONCEPTS

As medical practice became increasingly regulated during the course of the nineteenth and twentieth centuries, replacing the weak, fragmented and usually local forms of licensing and monopoly by guilds, royal colleges and medical faculties, responsible local and state authorities lacking the necessary resources and expertise frequently delegated regulatory power to representatives of the profession who were chosen in various ways. There were important exceptions like France where the elimination of traditional medical corporations left such authority in the hands of the state, which of course depended on its own medical experts for technical decisions (Weisz, 1995). The institutional basis of medical authority changed over time; it is probably fair to say that professional power oscillated, depending on the issues at stake, between academic and hospital elites and prominent rank-and-file practitioners, often outside the largest urban centres, organized in such representative bodies as the American or British Medical Association. At certain moments it reflected proximity to political power whether monarchical – the King's First Physician – or democratic. Such authority was based on certain common assumptions: the need to defend the economic self-interest of certified medical practitioners by limiting competition; that trained physicians represented the most authentic medical knowledge; the desire of politicians and administrators, physicians, and probably the educated public as well, to have a relatively safe health care environment based on practitioner competence. While there was also considerable pressure to keep the field of healing as open as possible, this could not withstand the movement to regulate healers and restrict the right to practice to those defined as competent. (Whether such restrictions were effective in practice is another matter.) Widespread agreement existed among key actors that 'scientific knowledge', however one defined science, was the most appropriate guarantee of competence and that such knowledge could be codified and tested on examinations.

This meant that authority to define both acceptable practitioners and acceptable practices were variably situated along several parameters. Whatever elements of group self-interest that might be involved in defining such parameters, arguments for medical authority had to be based on notions of the public good. At one end was authority to define who was allowed to be a medical practitioner; at the other was very fuzzy authority over actual medical practice (see Image 8.1). The two were only loosely if at all related. Moving to the vertical axis that defines objectives of authority, we can distinguish between concerns about the danger/risk that injury or even death that might result from poor medical practice and at the other end (or top) issues of efficiency, cost, control and even standardized practice that administrators and even physicians became increasingly concerned with. Such objectives emerged initially in large institutions like hospitals or public health programmes managing large populations, but gradually expanded to include individual private practice as this entered the public sphere through governmental financing or direct management. At the same time, authority over practice and practitioners combined informal norms, formal local or professional rules, and regulations and laws that had the authority of the state behind them.

Using this framework, we can say that the content of acceptable practice was for some time secondary to recognition of acceptable practitioners so that the formal credentials of practitioners served to guarantee a minimal level of good practice; these, combined with legal consequences for certain types of

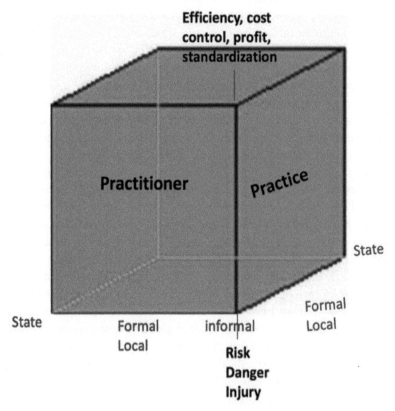

FIGURE 8.1: Graphic View of Traditional Medical Authority. Credit: George Weisz (Author).

malpractice and local beliefs and norms, constituted the basis for professional authority to practice medicine. This authority was usually granted by institutions of the profession, in partnership with political authorities (e.g. state legislatures) with some exceptions like France where the state played a more central role in partnership with medical elites. During the course of the twentieth century, governments became increasingly involved in defining competent practitioners and, eventually, acceptable practices. This was largely the consequence of health care's emergence as a 'public good' critically important to much of the population and paid for increasingly by public monies. As such it became the target of new kinds of public scrutiny. There have been two consequences of this long-term process. One has focused on efforts to control practice through rules – clinical practice guidelines and evidence-based medicine. Another has centred on the practitioner and made both training and certification increasingly long, intensive and deep.

SOME HISTORICAL BACKGROUND

It is well known by historians that medical practitioners since the Middle Ages were fragmented into separate self-regulating professions, each treating different conditions and social classes.[2] Physicians were university trained and specialized in internal diseases represented by physical signs like pulse or urine. Surgeons specialized in external conditions but also performed manual tasks like bleeding considered a method of balancing the humours; they significantly raised their status during the eighteenth century by taking on many of the trappings of learning and scholarship affected by physicians. Lower-status barber-surgeons combined two manual trades involving cutting. Finally, there were apothecaries, tradesmen who prepared pharmaceutical mixtures but frequently prescribed them as well. All these practitioners had their own guilds or colleges, and there was some rivalry and conflict among them. Aside from these recognized professions, there were also 'non-regulars' who were not part of legally organized guilds. Several kinds of non-regulars achieved considerable stature during the eighteenth century as they developed valued skills: these included oculists capable of couching cataracts and dentists who developed new techniques for making false teeth and dentures.

By the early twentieth century, many countries could boast relatively unified modern professions. These were not homogenous and divisions abounded; but partition into autonomous silos came more or less to an end. While it is difficult to summarize so many developments in numerous countries, it is fair to say that educational reform was at the heart of many of the changes that took place. This allowed new forms of stratification and division to come into being and transformed the traditional dynamics of the profession. In France, the process began early during the Revolutionary and Napoleonic periods with the central state creating and enforcing standardized training, certification and limited medical monopoly. In the US, after states in the 1830s and 1840s abolished their licensing laws in the name of Jacksonian democracy, freedom of practice was the rule until the last decades of the nineteenth century when a complex movement made up of elite medical schools, the American Medical Association (AMA), and state legislatures re-imposed state licensing controlled by the profession. In Canada, the process was simpler. As government spread from Quebec and Ontario throughout the thinly populated country, weak provincial authorities delegated professional certification and regulation to representatives of the profession called 'colleges', which gradually raised standards of medical training.

Britain probably came up with the most original solution: a state registry of physicians within a free market. Well into the nineteenth century, the division into separate professions of physicians, surgeons and apothecaries persisted. Each had its own system of licensing and governance. Rather than imposing legal unity, the reform act of 1858 created a medical register containing a single list of medical practitioners possessing one of the numerous recognized degrees. In exchange for this recognition, traditional occupations lost the limited monopolies that they had possessed previously. In other words, after 1858, anyone could practise medicine but patients could easily find out which practitioners had a state-certified licence with significant privileges attached. Here the monopoly was one of title rather than function. Anyone could practise as long as they did not claim to be a licensed healer. Gradually unification of recognized groups occurred as examining bodies got together to impose common educational standards.

The turn of the twentieth century seems to have been a critical period in this process of consolidation, rising status and increasing authority, engineered largely through education reform. We know this most clearly in the case of the US because the reforms associated with the Flexner Report (a symbol rather than cause of these changes) have received so much attention from defenders and critics alike. But similar processes were occurring in many Western nations. These educational reforms raised standards and reduced (usually temporarily) the number of newly certified practitioners, but also sought to improve the quality of those who made it through the training process. What made all this possible was the growing prestige of science as the arbiter of medical knowledge. Laboratory science in particular gained an important place in medical teaching and research, which forced medical schools to invest in equipment and specialized expertise, thus promoting the disappearance of less affluent institutions. Other factors included the growing popularity of alternative medicines, from homeopathy to osteopathy, which forced doctors and medical schools along with many institutions of alternative medicine to identify closely with the scientific foundations of medical knowledge. Playing a role as well was the prestige of foreign models of medical training, notably Germany for the basic sciences and Vienna for the medical specialities.[3]

Surviving schools received new funding, improved their teaching and raised recruitment standards. For a few years, at least, the well-trained physician was viewed as the guarantee of safety and rationality in medical practice, while providing a mechanism to control the market for healers. What destabilized the concept of the scientifically well-trained physician whose practices could be trusted was a new and rapidly expanding phenomenon: medical specialization. Specialization appeared among physicians in the 1830s and 1840s but did not achieve significant proportions until the early years of the twentieth century. From then on it continued expanding. By the mid-1930s, between forty and fifty-five per cent of all physicians in the great cities of Europe and North America called themselves specialists. The fact that they *could* all call themselves specialists was precisely the problem, for there was no accepted definition of a medical specialist. In some cases, general practitioners decided that they had sufficient experience with a condition or organ to function as specialists. In others, courses of four to six weeks allowed physicians to hang out shingles as specialists. Finally, there were the really well-trained (and angriest) specialists who spent years training in specialist hospital wards and resented the need to compete with individuals whom they viewed as unqualified.

One solution was to add a second form of training/certification to the MD degree designed especially for specialists. This was easier said than done because general practitioners were usually convinced that any new certification would transform them into second-class physicians unable to perform numerous procedures. Specialists who often resorted to general medicine (when patients needing specialist care were scarce) were in contrast afraid that the price of certification would be to close general practice to them. These issues were eventually ironed out and systems of specialist regulation and certification were gradually set up in most Western nations. The earliest ones were professionally organized and controlled (Germany 1923; Canada 1937; and in the United States continuous development of speciality boards during the 1920s and 1930s and up to the present). In both France and the United Kingdom, governmental systems were put into effect in 1947–8, as part of the creation of national health or health insurance systems; here one had to define specialists clearly, since they were paid more than general practitioners (Weisz, 2006).

By the 1960s, what guaranteed medical authority and competence of the physician were at least two levels of training and certification that were supposed to last an entire medical career. By then, however, this no longer seemed sufficient, partly because a growing research sector was constantly changing the knowledge base of medical practice and because government was now a major funder of health care, which had become organized around large bureaucratic institutions. This was true even in the United States, where government was by now paying for a significant share of health costs through the Veteran's Administration, Medicare and Medicaid. Issues of costs, safety, competence and appropriateness of care entered the public sphere in a major way. There were two sorts of responses to these developments.

THE RISE OF PRACTICE GUIDELINES

The first of these rested on efforts to standardize medical procedures.[4] Such standardization occurred at three interrelated levels. First, outside the traditional private relationship between doctor and patient were large-scale institutional settings for biomedical practices that were not necessarily controlled by physicians. There, the standardization of classifications, measures and procedures was perceived as a requirement for a variety of purposes, including the evaluation of outcomes, coordination of large-scale organizational activity and, later, third party payment. From the nineteenth century, public health was one such domain. Basic categories had to be defined and standardized in order to be useful, and doctors were constrained in a variety of ways – through standardized forms and/or instruments – to provide data that were uniform and comparable. Murderous epidemics definitely fell into the public sphere, and doctors as well as citizens were urged to act in the ways prescribed by public authorities who published instructions on how to deal with sporadic epidemics like cholera and yellow fever (Boston Board of Health, 1855). In the twentieth century, public health standards entered the world of clinical medicine as preventive public health expanded to the sphere of therapeutics through such mechanisms as programmes to treat sexually transmitted diseases, tuberculosis, infant mortality and cancer. Hospitals, which grew at a prodigious rate from the end of the nineteenth century, also generated demands for standardized organizational structures, practices and data collection.

Second, the results of medical research vastly complicated the world of medical practice and its regulation. Starting in the early twentieth century and accelerating after the Second World War, the expansion of research created new problems in translating this knowledge into better health care. Efforts to determine collectively the efficacy of so many new products and procedures intensified long-felt needs to standardize classification categories, instruments, measures and research protocols. Just as the standardization of public health eventually influenced medical practice, testing protocols frequently found their way into clinical practice in such technically sophisticated fields as cancer research. Finally, research has continued to produce new and increasingly complex procedures and instruments that cannot be used effectively without elaborate protocols that determine the actions of all health professionals.

Third, the private relationship between doctor and patient gradually became part of a public realm that was subject to new forms of bureaucratic control, rationality and knowledge. This was one consequence of an expanding governmental role as a provider or purchaser of health services and as a guarantor of the public's health. Much closer scrutiny of practices revealed extensive variation among institutions and practitioners. Such variation was viewed as increasingly problematic in the new medical order, an indication that someone was doing something wrong. This knowledge of variation was an outcome of the new information about health systems, the production of which itself generated yet greater need for standardized classifications, measures, practices and entities. The complex mechanisms introduced to monitor, evaluate and improve health care practices also demanded elaborate guidelines.

These pressures began to make themselves felt during the first third of the twentieth century. In the field of public health, many countries organized programmes to prevent and treat TB; later cancer-care programmes deployed new technologies that were complex and sometimes dangerous, notably the use of X-rays and radium, and that required guidelines and protocols for their safe and effective use (Dommann, 2006). New diagnostic laboratory tests also required elaborate instructions. The hospital efficiency movement sought to bring scientific management and industrial efficiency techniques to medicine (Reverby, 1981). The American College of Surgeons (ACS), created in 1917, served as a model for the other American specialities that followed the path of specialist certification. However, it also began standardizing practices through therapeutic evaluation, assessing cancer therapies on the basis of case records, and periodically publishing results (American College of Surgeons, 1931). In 1905, the American Medical Association (AMA) established the Council on Pharmacy and Chemistry to analyse the composition and quality of new drugs, with the results published in its *Journal of the American Medical Association*. These standards formed the basis for the revised federal drug regulation introduced during the 1930s (Marks, 1997; 2006). During the interwar years as well, the AMA also began evaluating the plethora of electrical instruments arriving on the market and tried to control diagnostic testing by recommending laboratories for doctors and hospitals to use (Weisz, 2006). The British government, by contrast, used a very different approach when establishing the Radium Trust and the Radium Commission in 1929, with the former buying radium on a large scale and the latter distributing it to hospitals. These bodies thus were able to tie the distribution of radium to the hospitals' adoption of specific standards of therapeutic practice and, in the process, had a major impact on the structure of cancer therapy nationally (Cantor, 2007).

After the Second World War, all aspects of the medical enterprise expanded dramatically, especially in the United States, which by then was the world's richest nation and the most profligate spender on health care. The expansion of both the public domains of medical practice and biomedical research, with their attendant multiplication of standards and protocols, made the standardization of medical procedures appear both feasible and imperative. The two were in fact intimately connected. One of the motivations for the development of the Diagnostic and Statistical Manual of Mental Disorders (DSM) III was to establish disease categories stable enough to be the subjects of fundable research (Healy, 1997; Wilson, 1993). Once established, however, these categories became fundamental to reimbursement procedures and thus to medical practice. The ongoing invention of complex technologies generated need for methods of assessment as well as protocols for their use.

From the mid-1970s on, the production of guidelines intensified and became subject to extensive comment and discussion. Between 1975 and 1984, guidelines were produced in many different countries, suggesting that the pressure for their spread cut across national borders. The United States nonetheless produced the majority of guidelines in an effort to come to terms with the rapid transformation of the American health care system (Weisz et al., 2007). New knowledge about practice variations, produced and analysed over several decades by John Wennberg, was especially influential in this process (Wennberg, 1979). He and others who questioned the appropriateness of certain medical practices challenged the notion of a universal medical science and raised serious quality issues (McPherson and Bunker, 2006). Such work was supplemented by questions raised by Archie Cochrane's influential book published in the UK, *Effectiveness and Efficiency*, about the scientific validity of many current and widely diffused medical procedures (Cochrane, 1972). Variation had come to be seen as a problem to be remedied. Despite considerable medical resistance to the introduction of 'cookbook medicine', by 1990 more than thirty-five physician organizations and speciality societies were reported to have developed guidelines; the AMA and the Council of Medical Specialty Societies had endorsed practice guidelines and were organizing speciality societies to set policy for their development; and academic medical centres had formed a research consortium on practice guidelines (Woolf, 1990). By the beginning of the next decade, guidelines were ubiquitous enough for the National Library of Medicine's PubMed to add to its list of publication types the categories 'Guidelines' in 1991 and 'Practice Guidelines' a year later. American guidelines were produced by a wide array of public health, research and advocacy institutions, as well as by numerous specialist medical societies. When the first articles on evidence-based medicine appeared in 1992, they gradually added a new level of formalization to guideline development, at least in certain circles, but they surfaced in a domain that was already well-established.

Although guideline development occurred first and foremost in the United States, it has been adopted in much of the Western world during the past thirty years. It is fair to say that we now live in a culture of clinical practice guidelines. This culture has been undermined by numerous critiques ranging from the influence of pharmaceutical companies on clinical trials and guideline development, to the technical inadequacies of many clinical trials, to the lack of real-world patients because of rigorous inclusion criteria. But it continues to prevail, despite numerous qualifications, doubts and concerns, because nothing more reliable has surfaced to replace it.

RECERTIFICATION AND REVALIDATION

As all this was going on, a related but independent process was underway. By the time a new speciality, family medicine, came into existence in 1969, mere speciality certification no longer seemed sufficient. Periodic 'recertification' was introduced as a requirement of specialist status in this field. If this largely reflected the uncertain status of a new speciality lacking a clearly defined knowledge base and out to prove its bona fides, the logic of the choice proved difficult to resist. As medicine's critics multiplied, its knowledge constantly expanded and changed, and political leaders were required to justify the monies they were pouring into health care, an increasingly defensive medical profession, or at least parts of it, felt compelled to respond. Marc Berg has documented how editorialists in medical journals during these decades framed the problem of the perceived inadequacies of medical practice (Berg, 1995; 1997). Consensus conferences, guidelines and EBM might be tools for solving these problems, but responsibility ultimately rested with the quality of physicians who applied or did not apply the results of these tools. Periodic recertification spread widely replacing the idea of lifelong competence following initial certification. It was gradually accepted by individual speciality boards and was adopted by all speciality boards in 1999, using cycles of seven to ten years. It was accompanied by continuing education programmes. Soon after, recertification was replaced by a new model known as 'maintenance of certification' (MOC), which was introduced during the early years of the twenty-first century. It includes demonstration of professional standing, lifelong learning, demonstration of cognitive expertise and demonstration of performance. Controversial reforms of MOC in 2014 compel many physicians to enrol in continuous, fee-paying certification programmes, completing tests every two years and performing practice improvement modules. Not surprisingly, 'some physicians view these tasks and costs as excessive' and opposition and criticism have been intense (Teirstein and Topol, 2015).

Not all physicians are subject to such recertification requirements. The forty per cent or so of American doctors who are not board certified are not bound by these regulations creating a rather large compliance gap. Nonetheless, periodic recertification, although not fully implemented, reflects a new ideal of competence and scientific authority, one that has to be constantly reviewed and upgraded in order to remain valid. The title of a 1989 article by Donald Berwick, one of the leading voices of the American quality of care movement, said it all: 'Continuous improvement as an ideal in health care' (1989). Mention of Berwick is a good place to remind readers that recertification/revalidation did not take place in a vacuum. During the 1990s, along with guidelines, EBM and recertification, Berwick was influential in advocating for greater safety in health care institutions, a position that was given wide publicity several years later when the Institute of Medicine published a major report suggesting that much unnecessary injury and death was caused by systemic and structural issues rather than individual mistakes (Kohn et al., 1999; Institute of Medicine, 2001). These and other movements of the period (the 'professionalism movement', for instance) fed into the larger search for greater guarantees of physician quality. In the words of one Canadian medical educator: 'Reading either the *Quality Chasm* or *To Err Is Human* . . . confirms the accumulated wisdom that holding a medical degree, a general license, or acquisition of a speciality certificate is insufficient evidence to ensure quality of care or patient safety' (Dauphenee, 2013).

Perhaps because Americans were spending so much more on health care than anyone else, or perhaps because American doctors on the whole earned considerably more than their colleagues elsewhere, the US was initially somewhat unique in its zeal to reform medical practice. Canadian doctors responded with noticeably less enthusiasm to the new professional norms. Certainly in 2004, the Canadian Adverse Events Study found considerable evidence of 'substantial burden of injury' among hospital patients and generated increased efforts to promote safety (Baker, 2014). However, provinces (health care is a provincial responsibility in Canada) have opted for mandatory continuing education programmes, without requiring re-examinations and recertification. Much the same is true in Europe. Several countries (Austria, Germany and Spain) focus on continuing medical education while others (Belgium, France and the Netherlands) also incorporate peer review (Merkur et al., 2008). In 2013, France introduced a more extensive system of continuing medical development in which doctors and all health personnel are required to analyse their own practices and then act to acquire or improve any knowledge or competence that is deemed to be weak (Da Silva, 2014). Austria, Germany and the Netherlands have all introduced professional development programmes of one sort or another (Dauphenee, 2013). The Medical Board of Australia (MBA) is currently examining the issue in order to work out a national strategy, but has already rejected the idea of revalidation (Flynn, 2017). In contrast, another agency, the Australia Health Practitioners Agency (AHPRA), is planning to introduce revalidation (Langlois, 2017).

Undoubtedly the most radical alternative to American-style recertification (managed by a professional body) was the validation procedure introduced in the UK in 2012 by government legislation. It involved:

- annual appraisal by a 'responsible officer'
- continuing professional development

- quality improvement activity
- reporting of significant events
- feedback from colleagues
- feedback from patients
- review of complaints and compliments.

The published *Instructions to Physicians* specified:

> Every five years, your responsible officer will make a recommendation to the GMC [General Medical Council] about your revalidation.
> The responsible officer will draw on the outcome of your annual appraisals, combined with any available information from the clinical governance systems of organisations in which you practise. . . .
> It is for the GMC to decide in each case whether you may continue to hold your licence to practise.

Making the process even more radical is the fact that the decisions made are not based exclusively on medical expertise. The GMC would have six lay and six medical members, all appointed following an independent appointments process. (However, there seems to be a second more directly professional revalidation path for specialists through one of the Royal Colleges.) The introduction of laypeople into this process, more than any other detail, seems responsible for the idea currently widespread in the medical and sociological literature that era of self-regulation (or 'club practice') of British medicine is now over. Authority, in this view, has devolved not so much to state control (although to that as well) but to 'stakeholder' control, for the chief barrier to revalidation is alienating the patients and colleagues who now report on physician practice. As was the case with EBM, criticism has decreased as it has become clear that implementation is less demanding than regulations suggest. And inevitably, efforts are being made to develop standardized metrics to evaluate performance (Van der Meulen et al., 2017).

What lies behind these radical changes? Issues of safety have emerged in the UK, as in the US, with the added piquancy of several well-publicized malpractice scandals, like that of the serial murderer Harold Shipman and that of the Royal Bristol Infirmary. As in the US, demands by consumers and administrators for greater transparency and accountability play a large part in these reforms. As in the US as well, there is support from parts of the profession as it struggles to adjust to new conditions while retaining as much autonomy as possible. It is also possible that American models have come into play and influence British and European medical elites more generally. And it is likely that as much as ensuring safety, these reforms are linked to desire for standardization, an end to practice variation, and the aspiration to bring order and functional rationality to unwieldy health care institutions that have emerged piecemeal over several centuries and are now supposed to be administered as parts of 'systems'.

CONCLUDING THOUGHTS

Periodic revalidation and maintenance of certification (MOC) are discussed frequently and passionately in the medical literature. But unlike EBM and clinical practice guidelines, they have not broken out of the narrow professional sphere to attract much attention from social scientists. This is not entirely surprising, since it is not easy actually to find details of how these programmes are working in practice as opposed to how they are *supposed* to function. But part of the story may be that EBM has been far more interesting to social scientists because it appears to represent an epistemological rupture replacing one form of authority – expertise/experience – with another more 'objective' one based on RCTs and meta-analyses. Indeed, its proponents initially characterized it (quite naively) as a new 'paradigm'. Periodic revalidation, in contrast, seems almost a natural continuation of developments in medical training that have been going on for two centuries: the accretion of new criteria and tests defining competence. Such continuity has indeed been stressed by some of its leading exponents (Mcgaghie, 2013). It also appears to be a common-sense response to the constant evolution of medical knowledge and practices that seem to render initial training quickly obsolete. But this is only part of the story. Like EBM, MOC and revalidation allow both the profession and health care administrators to try to get out in front of problems and undercut potential criticism. However, there is also something about this quest for never-ending self-improvement that runs deeper and that reflects a medical self-image rooted not just in competence but in what I can only call humanitarian idealism, which has a long history in medical rhetoric (Weisz, 1987). Functionalist sociologists of the 1940s and 1950s took this claim seriously enough to make social altruism one of the defining features of modern professions of which medicine was the exemplar (Parsons, 1949). While this type of sociology was soon replaced by more critical and dynamic approaches to professions, the tradition of humanitarian care remains pertinent for physicians. It is at the core of the emphasis on 'altruism' as the first principle in the widely adopted Charter on Medical Professionalism: 'This principle is based on a dedication to serving the interest of the patient. Altruism contributes to the trust that is central to the physician–patient relationship' (Medical Professionalism Project, 2002). This has remained a central concern within the larger Professionalism movement, despite cogent critiques of its applicability to both medical training and professional identity (Harris, 2017).

This last point raises an interesting issue. Reading the literature on revalidation, I am struck by how little reference there is to EBM. We are talking about a wide-ranging movement with equally wide-ranging motives, and in some cases, little is said because the link is probably self-evident; after all, what is going to define inadequacy or improvement in practice, if not EBM-based guidelines? But in other cases, the role of peers and patients in the UK and other countries suggests a rather different kind of logic in which professional collegiality and patient satisfaction play far more important roles than guidelines. This is reflected in the search for new metrics of evaluation. A study of INCEPT: A Multisource Feedback Tool for Professional Performance is being tested focused on 'professional attitude', 'patient-centeredness' and 'organization and (self)-management' (van der Meulen, 2017). A survey of the subject internationally argued years ago that 'there is a move from continuing medical education (or clinical update) to continuing professional development, including medical, managerial, social, and personal skills' (Peck et al., 2000). Clearly in many contexts, continuing medical education and revalidation may well be functioning on a rather different register than EBM. One potential source for this shift is elite medical schools, which have for the past century combined training with research, care with science (Dunn and Jones, 2010). Certainly from 1945 to the end of the century, it was the research function that was more valued in prestigious medical schools. This dynamic began to change during the last decades of the twentieth century, partly because influential groups of patients were demanding a different kind of care, but also because the training of primary care physicians became a political priority almost everywhere. Training in primary care has traditionally been more attuned to developing skills and human relations rather than advancing research, an area where domains like family medicine have had some difficulty in competing with specialities (Post et al., 2012). As primary care has taken on a larger role in medical education, its pedagogical values have infiltrated the curriculum.

EBM and MOC have several things in common, aside from the common aspiration to improve medical practice. Both can be seen as efforts to maintain some degree of professional control over definitions of credentials and quality of practice. It is true that EBM has shifted somewhat the balance of power within the medical profession away from traditional elites to new centres of expertise while the British version of revalidation gives some influence to patients and to managers. But MOC in particular retains decision-making within the bounds of the organized profession. It is an alternative to outside administrative or political control. As one article that proposes to make MOC assessments less burdensome and more effective has concluded: 'We believe that protecting the integrity of a peer-defined, discipline-specific credential is not the role of the government, health care delivery systems, or payers – it belongs to those of us who practice the discipline, maintaining highly specialized knowledge and demonstrating that we have done so' (Baron and Braddock, 2016: 217). To the extent that all such programmes now emphasize patient satisfaction, they constitute an alternative way of dealing with the consumer culture that has patients rating doctors in the same way that they rate restaurants and electronics (Tomes, 2016).

Another feature that EBM and MOC share is reliance on faith or, to be less provocative, common-sense thinking rather than on real evidence. As critics have long stated in the case of EBM and more recently revalidation, neither has ever been reliably demonstrated to improve medical outcomes (Scallan, 2016). This could prove eventually to be a problem for EBM, whose raison d'être is evidence. In the case of revalidation or MOC, this may be less important. Medical authority, whatever its current status in comparison to the past, is in the final analysis not based on quantifiable results of physician practice but rather on public perceptions that physicians are the best-trained and most knowledgeable experts in maintaining health and curing disease. (The current COVID pandemic, as it is playing out in the USA, provides a particularly vivid example of just how critical trust in authorities can be during a crisis, where evidence accumulates slowly, uncertainly and sporadically.) The perception of medical competence, like the claim that the physician's commitment to patient well-being is total, is made concrete and substantial by a visible and never-ending quest for self-improvement.

NOTES

1. The most influential (if hardly original) version of this argument is Starr's *The Social Transformation of American Medicine: The Rise of a Sovereign Profession and the Making of a Vast Industry*.
2. What follows summarizes well-known developments that have been described in far too many works to be cited here.
3. On these changes internationally, see Bonner's *Becoming a Physician: Medical Education in Britain, France, Germany, and the United States, 1750–1945*.
4. This section draws heavily on Weisz et al.'s 'The emergence of clinical practice guidelines', *The Milbank Quarterly*.

BIBLIOGRAPHY

INTRODUCTION

Ackerknecht, E. (1955), *Short History of Medicine*. Baltimore: Johns Hopkins University Press.

Adams, A. (2007), *Medicine by Design: The Architect and the Modern Hospital, 1893–1943*. Minneapolis: University of Minnesota Press.

Biehl, J. and A. Petryna (eds.) (2013), *When People Come First: Critical Studies in Global Health*. Princeton: Princeton University Press.

Brandt, A. (1991), 'Emerging themes in the history of medicine', *The Milbank Quarterly*, 69: 199–214.

Braunstein, J.-F. (2010), 'Histoire et philosophie de la médicine', *Archives de philosophie*, 73: 579–83.

Burke, P. (2004), *What is Cultural History?* London: Polity Press.

Bynum, W. F. (1994), *Science and the Practice of Medicine in the Ninetieth Century*. New York: Cambridge University Press.

Canguilhem, G. (2012), *Writings on Medicine*. New York: Fordham University Press.

Cooter, R. (1985), *The Cultural Meaning of Popular Science*. Cambridge: Cambridge University Press.

Cooter, R. (2007), '"After death/after life": the social history of medicine in post-postmodernity', *Social History of Medicine*, 20: 441–64.

Cooter, R. with Stein, C. (2013), *Writing History in the Age of Biomedicine*. New Haven: Yale University Press.

Fanon, F. (1994 [1965]), *A Dying Colonialism*. New York: Grove Press.

Farmer, P. (1992), *AIDS and Accusation: Haiti and the Geography of Blame*. Berkeley: University of California Press.

Fee, E. (1983), *Women and Health: The Politics of Sex in Medicine*. London: Routledge.

Fee, E. and D. M. Fox (1988), *AIDS: The Burdens of History*. Berkeley: University of California Press.

Forrester, J. (2017), *Thinking in Cases*. London: Polity.

Golinski, J. (1998), *Making Natural Knowledge: Constructivism and the History of Science*. New York: Cambridge University Press.

Good, B. J. (1994), *Medicine, Rationality, and Experience: An Anthropological Perspective*. New York: Cambridge University Press.

Greene, J. (2008), *Prescribing by Numbers: Drugs and the Definition of Disease*. Baltimore: Johns Hopkins University Press.

Hayward, R. (2005), '"Much exaggerated": the end of the history of medicine', *Journal of Contemporary History*, 40: 167–78.

Hunt, N. R. (1999), *A Colonial Lexicon: Of Birth Ritual, Medicalization, and Mobility in the Congo*. Durham: Duke University Press.

Iggers, G. G. (1997), *Historiography in the Twentieth Century: From Scientific Objectivity to the Postmodern Challenge*. Hanover: Wesleyan University Press.

Illich, I. (1976), *Limits to Medicine: Medical Nemesis, the Expropriation of Health*. London: Marion Boyars Publishers.

Jain, S. L. (2013), *Malignant: How Cancer Becomes Us*. Berkeley: University of California Press.

Keller, R. C. (2015), *Fatal Isolation: The Devastating Paris Heat Wave of 2013*. Chicago: University of Chicago Press.

King, C. R. (1991), 'The Historiography of Medical History: From Great Men to Archaeology', *Bulletin of the New York Academy of Medicine*, 67(5): 407–28.

Lederer, S. E. (1997), *Subjected to Science: Human Experimentation in America Before the Second World War*. Baltimore: Johns Hopkins University Press.

Lindenbaum, S. (1978), *Kuru Sorcery: Disease and Danger in the New Guinea Highlands*. Palo Alto: Mayfield Publishing.

Livingston, J. (2012), *Improvising Medicine: An African Oncology Ward in an Emerging Cancer Epidemic*. Durham: Duke University Press.

Löwy, L. (2011), 'Historiography of biomedicine: "bio" "medicine" and in between', *Isis*, 102(1): 116–22.

Marks, H. (1997), *The Progress of Experiment: Science and Therapeutic Reform in the United States, 1900–1990*. New York: Cambridge University Press.

Martin, E. (1987), *The Woman in the Body: A Cultural Analysis of Reproduction*. Boston: Beacon Press.

Nguyen, V-K. (2010), *The Republic of Therapy: Triage and Sovereignty in West Africa's Time of AIDS*. Durham: Duke University Press.

Packard, R. M. (2016), *A History of Global Health: Interventions into the Lives of Other Peoples*. Baltimore: Johns Hopkins University Press.

Porter, D. (1999), *Health, Civilization, and the State*. London: Routledge.

Porter, R. (1985), 'The Patient's View: Doing Medical History from Below', *Theory and Society*, 14(2): 175–98.

Porter, R. (1997), *The Greatest Benefit to Mankind: A Medical History of Humanity*. New York: Norton.

Porter, R. (ed.) (2006), *The Cambridge History of Medicine*. New York: Cambridge University Press.

River, W. H. R. (2001 [1924]), *Medicine, Magic, and Religion*. London: Routledge.

Rose, N. (2007), 'Beyond medicalisation', *The Lancet*, 369: 700–2.

Rosen, G. (1949), 'Levels of Integration in Medical Historiography: A Review' *Journal of the History of Medicine and Allied Health Sciences*, 4(4): 460–7.

Rosen, G. (2015), *A History of Public Health*. Baltimore: Johns Hopkins University Press.

Rosenberg, C. (1998), 'Pathologies of progress: the idea of civilization as risk', *Bulletin of the History of Medicine*, 72: 714–30.

Rosenberg, C. (2007), *Our Present Complaint: American Medicine, Then and Now*. Baltimore: Johns Hopkins University Press.

Rosner, D. and G. Markowitz (2006), *Deadly Dust: Silicosis and the Ongoing Struggle to Protect Workers' Health*. Ann Arbor: University of Michigan Press.

Sigerist, H. E. (1960), *On the Sociology of Medicine*. New York: MD Publications.

Sigerist, H. E. (1994), *American Medicine*. New York: W. W. Norton.

Sigerist, H. E. (2010), *Henry E. Sigerist: Correspondence with Welch, Cushing, Garrison, and Ackerknecht*. Bern: Peter Lang.

Sigerist, H. E. (2018), *Civilization and Disease*. Ithaca: Cornell University Press.

Starr, P. (1984), *The Social Transformation of American Medicine: The Rise of a Sovereign Profession and the Making of a Vast Industry*. New York: Basic Books.

Stevens, R. (1989), *In Sickness and in Wealth: American Hospitals in the Twentieth-Century*. Baltimore: Johns Hopkins University Press.

Stevens, R. (1998), *American Medicine and the Public Interest*. Berkeley: University of California Press.

Tomes, N. (1998), *The Gospel of Germs: Men, Women, and the Microbe in American Life*. Cambridge: Harvard University Press.

Tone, A. (2001), *Devices and Desires: A History of Contraceptives in America*. New York: Hill and Wang.

Treichler, P. A. (1999), *How to Have Theory in an Epidemic: Cultural Chronicles of AIDS*. Durham: Duke University Press.

Weisz, G. (2005), *Divide and Conquer: A Comparative History of Medical Specialization*. New York: Oxford University Press.

Weisz, G. (2014), *Chronic Disease in the Twentieth Century: A History*. Baltimore: Johns Hopkins University Press.

Worsley, P. (1982), 'Non-Western medical systems', *Annual Review of Anthropology*, 11: 315–48.

1. ENVIRONMENT

Anderson, W. H. (2004), 'Natural histories of infectious disease: ecological vision in twentieth-century biomedical science', *Osiris*, 19: 39–61.

Aronowitz, R. (2012), 'The rise and fall of the Lyme disease vaccines: a cautionary tale for risk interventions in American medicine and public health', *Milbank Quarterly*, 90(2): 250–77.

Barbour, A. (2015), *Lyme Disease: Why It's Spreading, How It Makes You Sick, and What to Do about It*. Baltimore: Johns Hopkins University Press.

Baum, D. (2016), 'Legalize it all: how to win the war on drugs', *Harpers* 1 April.

Bersani, L. (1995), *Homos*. Cambridge, MA: Harvard University Press.

Bersani, L. (2009), *Is the Rectum a Grave? and Other Essays*. Chicago: University of Chicago Press.

Bourgois, P. (1995), *In Search of Respect: Selling Crack in El Barrio*. New York and Cambridge: Cambridge University Press.

Bourgois, P. (1998), 'Just another night in a shooting gallery', *Theory, Culture and Society*, 15(2): 37–66.

Bourgois, P. (2009), *Righteous Dopefiend*. Berkeley: University of California Press.

Bourgois, P. et al. (1997), 'Social misery and the sanctions of substance abuse: confronting HIV risk among homeless heroin addicts in San Francisco', *Social Problems*, 44(2): 155–73.

Brandt, A. M. (1988), 'AIDS in historical perspective: four lessons from the history of sexually transmitted disease', *American Journal of Public Health*, 78: 367–71.

Carson, R. (2002), *Silent Spring*. New York: Houghton Mifflin.

Cohen, C. (1999), *The Boundaries of Blackness: AIDS and the Breakdown of Black Politics*. Chicago: University of Chicago Press.

Comfort, L. et al. (1999), 'Reframing disaster policy: the global evolution of vulnerable communities', *Environmental Hazards*, 1: 39–44.

Conis, E. (2014), *Vaccine Nation: America's Changing Relationship with Immunization*. Chicago: University of Chicago Press.

Craddock, S. (2000), *City of Plagues: Disease, Poverty, and Deviance in San Francisco*. Minneapolis: University of Minnesota Press.

Cromley, E. K. et al. (1998), 'Residential setting as a risk factor for Lyme disease in a hyperendemic region', *American Journal of Epidemiology*, 147(5): 472–7.

Cunningham, A. (1992), 'Transforming plague: the laboratory and the identity of infectious disease', in Andrew Cunningham and Perry Williams (eds.), *The Laboratory Revolution in Medicine*, Cambridge: Cambridge University Press, pp. 209–44.

DiChiro, G. (1995), 'Nature as community: the convergence of environment and social justice', in William Cronon (ed.), *Uncommon Ground: Toward Reinventing Nature*, New York: W.W. Norton, pp. 298–320.

Echenberg, M. (2002), 'Pestis redux: the initial years of the third bubonic plague pandemic, 1894–1901', *Journal of World History*, 13: 429–49.

Echenberg, M. (2007), *Plague Ports: The Global Urban Impact of Bubonic Plague 1894–1901*. New York: New York University Press.

Edlow, J. (2003), *Bull's Eye: Unraveling the Medical Mystery of Lyme Disease*. New Haven: Yale University Press.

Essex, M. and P. Kanki (1988), 'The origins of the AIDS virus', *Scientific American*, 259: 44–51.

Faria, N. R. et al. (2014), 'HIV epidemiology: the early spread and epidemic ignition of HIV-1 in human populations', *Science*, 346(6205): 56–61.

Folkers, K. M. (2016), 'Zika: The Millennials' S.T.D.?' *The New York Times*, 20 August.

Freed, L. J. (2010), Networks of (colonial) power: roads in French Central Africa after World War I, *History and Technology*, 26: 203–23.

Garrett, L. (1995), *The Coming Plague: Newly Emerging Diseases in a World Out of Balance*. New York: Penguin.

Giles-Vernick, T. et al. (2013), 'Social history, biology and the emergence of HIV in colonial Africa', *Journal of African History*, 54(1): 11–30.

Hahn, B. and G. M. Shaw (2000), 'AIDS as a zoonosis: scientific and public health implications', *Science*, 287(5453): 607–14.

Jones, S. D. (2011), 'Hunting the *Hant'a*: the implications of sylvatic plague for public health', paper presented at the workshop *Re-thinking the History of Health, Disease, and Medicine in Global Perspective*, at University of Oxford, 26 September.

Keller, R. C. (2015), *Fatal Isolation: The Devastating Paris Heat Wave of 2003*. Chicago: University of Chicago Press.

Kilcup, K. L. (2013), *Fallen Forests: Emotion, Embodiment, and Ethics in American Women's Environmental Writing, 1781–1924*. Athens: University of Georgia Press.

Klass, P. (2017), 'Too clean for our children's good?' *New York Times*, 17 April.

Landecker, H. (2011), 'Food as exposure: nutritional epigenetics and the new metabolism', *BioSocieties*, 6(2): 167–94.

Landecker, H. and A. Panofsky (2013), 'From social structure to gene regulation, and back: a critical introduction to environmental epigenetics for sociology', *Annual Review of Sociology*, 39: 333–57.

Langston, N. (2010), *Toxic Bodies: Hormone Disruptors and the Legacy of DES*. New Haven: Yale University Press.

Lappé, M. (2016), 'The maternal body as environment in autism science', *Social Studies of Science*, 46(5): 675–700.

Latour, B. (1988), *The Pasteurization of France*, translated by Alan Sheridan and John Law. Cambridge, MA: Harvard University Press.

Lederer, S. E. (2008), *Flesh and Blood: Organ Transplantation and Blood Transfusion in 20th-Century America*. Oxford: Oxford University Press.

Livingston, J. (2012), *Improvising Medicine: An African Oncology Ward in an Emerging Cancer Epidemic*. Durham: Duke University Press.

Maugh, T. H. (1978), 'Cancer and environment: Higginson speaks out', *Science*, 205(4413): 1363–6.

McNeill, W. H. (1976), *Plagues and Peoples*. New York: Anchor; Summers, W. (2012), *The Great Manchurian Plague of 1910–1911: Geopolitics of an Epidemic Disease*. New Haven: Yale University Press.

Milgram, S. (1970), 'The experience of living in cities', *Science*, 167(3924): 1461–8.

Mitman, G. (2005), 'In search of health: landscape and disease in American environmental history', *Environmental History*, 10: 184–209.

Mitman, G. (2007), *Breathing Space: How Allergies Shape Our Lives and Landscapes*. New Haven: Yale University Press.

Moore, K. (2016), *Radium Girls*. New York: Simon and Schuster.

Murphy, M. (2006), *Sick Building Syndrome and the Problem of Uncertainty: Environmental Politics, Technoscience, and Women Workers*. Durham: Duke University Press.

Nash, L. (2006), *Inescapable Ecologies: A History of Environment, Disease, and Knowledge*. Berkeley: University of California Press.

Nixon, R. (2011), *Slow Violence and the Environmentalism of the Poor*. Cambridge, MA: Harvard University Press.

Nixon, R. (2014), 'The Anthropocene: the promise and pitfalls of an epochal idea', *Edge effects*. http://edgeeffects.net/anthropocene-promise-and-pitfalls (accessed 12 June 2017).

Pasternak, J. (2011), *Yellow Dirt: A Poisoned Land and the Betrayal of the Navajos*. New York: Free Press.

Patz, J. A., P. Daszak, G. M. Tabor, A. A. Aguirre, M. Pearl, J. Epstein, N. D. Wolfe, A. M. Kilpatrick, J. Foufopoulos, D. Molyneux, D. J. Bradley and Members of the Working Group on Land Use Change and Disease Emergence (2004), 'Unhealthy landscapes: policy recommendations on land use change and infectious disease emergence', *Environmental Health Perspectives*, 101: 1092–8.

Patz, J. A., S. H. Olson, C. K. Uejio and H. K. Gibbs (2008), 'Disease emergence from climate and land use change', *Medical Clinics of North America*, 92: 1473–91.

Pepin, J. (2011), *The Origin of AIDS*. Cambridge: Cambridge University Press.

Petryna, A. (2002), *Life Exposed: Biological Citizenship after Chernobyl*. Princeton: Princeton University Press.

Pollan, M. (2013), 'Some of my best friends are germs', *New York Times Magazine*, 15 May.

Proctor, R. N. (1995), *Cancer Wars: How Politics Shapes What We Know and Don't Know about Cancer*. New York: Basic Books.

Proctor, R. N. (1999), *The Nazi War on Cancer*. Princeton: Princeton University Press.

Proctor, R. N. (2012), *Golden Holocaust: Origins of the Cigarette Catastrophe and the Case for Abolition*. Berkeley: University of California Press.

Reagan, L. J. (2011), 'Representations and reproductive hazards of Agent Orange', *Journal of Law, Medicine, and Ethics*, 39: 1.

Robins, L. N. et al. (2010), 'Vietnam veterans three years after Vietnam: how our study changed our view of heroin', *American Journal of Addiction*, 19(3): 203–11.

Rome, A. (2001), *The Bulldozer in the Countryside: Suburban Sprawl and the Rise of American Environmentalism*. Cambridge: Cambridge University Press.

Rosenberg, C. (1998), 'Pathologies of progress: the idea of civilization as risk', *Bulletin of the History of Medicine*, 72: 714–30.

Rosner, D. and G. Markowitz (2006), *Deadly Dust: Silicosis and the Ongoing Struggle to Protect Workers' Health*. Ann Arbor: University of Michigan Press.

Sharp, P. M. and B. H. Hahn, B (2011), 'Origins of HIV and the AIDS pandemic', *Cold Spring Harbor Perspectives in Medicine*, 1(1): 1–22.

Shilts, R. (1987), *And the Band Played On*. New York: St. Martin's Press.

Shostak, S. (2013), *Exposed Science: Genes, the Environment, and the Politics of Population Health*. Berkeley: University of California Press.

Simpson, W. J. R. (1905), *A Treatise on Plague*. Cambridge: Cambridge University Press.

Sinhal, K. (2011), 'Cancer cases in Bhopal have tripled: ICMR study', *Times of India*, 27 February.

Stefansson, V. (1960), *Cancer: Diseases of Civilization? An Anthropological and Historical Study*. New York: Hill and Wang.

Steinberg, T. (2001), *Acts of God: The Unnatural History of Natural Disaster*. Oxford: Oxford University Press.

Swanson, M. W. (1977), 'The sanitation syndrome: bubonic plague and urban native policy in the Cape Colony, 1900–1909', *Journal of African Studies*, 18(3): 387–410.

Treichler, P. (1999), *How to Have Theory in an Epidemic: Cultural Chronicles of AIDS*. Durham: Duke University Press.

Vann, M. G. (2003), 'Of rats, rice, and race: the great Hanoi rat massacre, an episode in French colonial history', *French Colonial History*, 4: 191–203.

Walkowitz, J. (1992), *City of Dreadful Delight: Narratives of Sexual Danger in late Victorian London*. Chicago: University of Chicago Press.

Watkins, E. S. (2016), 'Reconceiving the pill: from revolutionary therapeutic to lifestyle drug', in Jeremy Greene, Elizabeth Siegel Watkins and Flurin Condrau (eds.), *Therapeutic Revolutions: Pharmaceuticals and Social Change in the Twentieth Century*, Chicago: University of Chicago Press, pp. 43–64.

Weiss, R. A. and R. W. Wrangham (1999), 'From *pan* to pandemic', *Nature*, 397: 385–6.

Wolfe, N. D. et al. (2005), 'Bushmeat hunting, deforestation, and prediction of zoonotic disease emergence', *Emerging Infectious Diseases*, 11(12): 1822–7.

Worboys, M. (2000), *Spreading Germs: Disease Theories and Medical Practice in Britain, 1865–1900*. Cambridge: Cambridge University Press.

World Health Organization (2008), *Global Burden of Disease: 2004 Update*. Geneva: WHO Press.

2. FOOD

Ames, B. (1999), 'Micronutrient deficiencies: a major cause of DNA damage', *Annals of the New York Academy of Science*, (October): 87–106.

Bestor, T. C. (2004), *Tsukiji: The Fish Market at the Center of the World*. Berkeley: University of California Press.

Carpenter, D. (2014), *Reputation and Power: Organizational Image and Pharmaceutical Regulation at the FDA*. Princeton: Princeton University Press.

Crider, K., L. Bailey, and R. Berry (2011), 'Folic acid food fortification – its history, effect, concerns, and future directions', *Nutrients*, 3(3): 370–84.

Daemmrich, A. and M. E. Bowden (2005), 'A rising drug industry', *Chemical and Engineering News*, 85(25): 28–42.

Dumit, J. (2012), *Drugs for Life: How Pharmaceutical Companies Define Our Health*. Durham: Duke University Press.

Dupuis, M. (2015), *Dangerous Digestion: The Politics of American Dietary Advice*. Berkeley: University of California Press.

Friedberg, S. (2004), *French Bean and Food Scares: Culture and Commerce in an Anxious Age*. New York: Oxford University Press.

Gilman, S. L. (2008), *Diets and Dieting: A Cultural Encyclopedia*. London: Routledge.

Greene, J. (2007), *Prescribing by Numbers: Drugs and the Definition of Disease*. Baltimore: Johns Hopkins University Press.

Guthman, J. (2011), *Weighing In: Obesity, Food Justice, and the Limits of Capitalism*. Berkeley: University of California Press.

Hargrove, J. (2006), 'History of the Calorie in Nutrition', *Journal of Nutrition*, 136: 2957–61.

Hilts, P. J. (2004), *Protecting America's Health: The FDA, Business, and One Hundred Years of Regulation*. Chapel Hill: University of North Carolina Press.

Holmes, S. (2013), *Fresh Fruit, Broken Bodies: Migrant Farmworkers in the United States*. Berkeley: University of California Press.

Horton, S. (2016), *They Leave Their Kidneys in the Field: Illness, Injury, and Illegality Among American Farmworkers*. Berkeley: University of California Press.

Junod, S. (2001), 'Folic acid fortification: fact and folly', Selections From FDLI Update Series on FDA History series on https://www.fda.gov/aboutfda/whatwedo/history/productregulation/selectionsfromfdliupdateseriesonfdahistory (accessed on 30 July 2017).

Kimura, A. (2013), *Hidden Hunger: Gender and The Politics of Smarter Foods*. Ithaca: Cornell University Press.

Lakoff, A. (2006), *Pharmaceutical Reason: Knowledge and Value in Global Psychiatry*. New York: Cambridge University Press.

Landeker, H. (2011), 'Food as exposure: nutritional epigenetics and the new metabolism', *BioSocieties*, 6: 167–94.

Langlitz, N. (2009), 'Pharmacovigilance and post-black market surveillance', *Social Studies of Science*, 39(3): 395–420.

Mintz, S. (1982), *Sweetness and Power: The Place of Sugar in Modern History*. New York: Penguin Books.

Mudry, J. (2009), *Measured Meals: Nutrition in America*. Albany: SUNY Press.

Muenster, D. (2015), '"Ginger is a gamble": crop booms, rural uncertainty, and the neoliberalization of agriculture in South India', *Focaal*, 71: 100–13.

Nestle, M. (2002), *Food Politics: How the Food Industry Influences Nutrition and Health*. Berkeley: University of California Press.

Nestle, M. (2003), *Safe Food: The Politics of Food Safety*. Berkeley: University of California Press.

Paxson, H. (2014), 'Interlude: microbiopolitics', in Eben Kirksey (ed.), *The Multispecies Salon*, Durham: Duke University Press.

Petryna, A. (2005), 'Ethical variability: drug development and globalizing clinical trials', *American Ethnologist*, 32(2): 183–97.

Solomon, H. (2016), *Metabolic Living: Food, Fat, and the Absorption of Illness in India*. Durham: Duke University Press.

Weisz, G. (2014), *Chronic Disease in the Twentieth Century: A History*. Baltimore: Johns Hopkins University Press.

Zhan, M. (2009), *Other Worldly: Making Chinese Medicine through Transnational Frames*. Durham: Duke University Press.

3. DISEASE

Anderson, W. (2006), *Colonial Pathologies: American Tropical Medicine, Race, and Hygiene in the Philippines*. Durham: Duke University Press.

Aronowitz, R. (2007), *Unnatural History: Breast Cancer and American Society*. New York: Cambridge University Press.

Bayer, R. (1981), *Homosexuality and American Psychiatry: The Politics of Diagnosis*. New York: Basic Books.

Becker, H. (1963), *Outsiders: The Sociology of Deviance*. New York: Glencoe.

Berger, P. and T. Luckmann (1966), *The Social Construction of Reality: A Treatise in the Sociology of Knowledge*. Garden City: Doubleday.

Best, C. (1963), *Selected Papers of Charles Best*. Toronto: University of Toronto Press.

Birn, A.-E. and A. Solórzano (1997), 'The hook of hookworm: public health and the politics of eradication in Mexico', in A. Cunningham and B. Andrews (eds.), *Western Medicine as Contested Knowledge*, Manchester: Manchester University Press/New York: St. Martin's Press, pp. 147–71.

Bliss, M. (1983), *The Discovery of Insulin*. Chicago: University of Chicago Press.

Boutayeb, A. (2006), 'The double burden of communicable and non-communicable diseases in developing countries', *Transactions of the Royal Society of Tropical Medicine & Hygiene*, 100(3): 191–9.

Brandt, A. M. (1985), *No Magic Bullet: A Social History of Venereal Disease*. New York: Oxford University Press.

Brandt, A. M. (2007), *The Cigarette Century: The Rise, Fall, and Deadly Persistence of the Product That Defined America*. New York: Basic Books.

Bygbjerg, I. C. (2012), 'Double burden of noncommmunicable and infectious diseases in developing countries', *Science*, 337(6101): 1499–1501.

Caduff, C. (2015), *The Pandemic Perhaps: Dramatic Events in a Public Culture of Danger*. Berkeley: University of California Press.

Canguilhem, G. (1989), *The Normal and the Pathological*. New York: Zone Books.

Childs, B. F. (1995), 'The logic of disease', in C. R. Scriver, A. L. Beaudet, W. S. Sly and D. Valle (eds.), *The Metabolic and Molecular Basis of Inherited Disease, 7th edition*. New York: McGraw-Hill.

Conrad, P. (1975), 'The discovery of hyperkinesis: notes on the medicalization of deviant behavior', *Social Problems*, 23(1): 12–21.

Cooper, D. G. (1967), *Psychiatry and Anti-Psychiatry*. London: Paladin.

Cruickshank, P. J. (2011), *The Teleology of Care: Reinventing International Health, 1968–1989*. Cambridge, MA: Harvard University, unpublished PhD dissertation.

Cueto, M. (1995), 'The cycles of eradication: Rockefeller Foundation and Latin American public health', in P. Weindling (ed.), *International Health and Welfare Organizations between the First and Second World Wars*. Cambridge: Cambridge University Press, pp. 179–202.

Davis, D. (2007), *The Secret History of the War on Cancer*. New York: Basic Books.

Debru, C. (2002), 'From nineteenth century ideas on reduction in physiology to non-reductive explanations in twentieth-century biochemistry', in M. H. V. Regenmortel and D. L. Hull (eds.), *Promises and limits of reductionism in the biomedical sciences*, Philadelphia: John Wiley & Sons. pp. 35–46.

Desjarlais, R., L. Eisenberg, B. Good and A. Kleinman (1996), *World Mental Health: Problems and Priorities in Low-Income Countries*. Oxford: Oxford University Press.

Dooley, K. E. and R. E. Chaisson (2009), 'Tuberculosis and diabetes mellitus: convergence of two epidemics', *Lancet Infectious Diseases*, 9: 737.

Dubòs, R. (1952), *The White Plague: Tuberculosis, Man, and Society*. New York: Little, Brown, and Company.

Dumit, J. (2012), *Drugs for Life: How Pharmaceutical Companies Define Our Health*. Durham: Duke University Press.

Ehrenreich, B. and D. English (1978), *Complaints and Disorders: The Sexual Politics of Sickness*. Old Westbury: The Feminist Press.

Eisenberg, L. and A. Kleniman (1981), *The Relevance of Social Science for Medicine*. Dordrecht: D. Reidel.

Epstein, S. (1993), *Impure Science: AIDS, Activism, and the Politics of Knowledge*. Berkeley: University of California Press.

Escobar, A. (1995), *Encountering Development: The Making and Unmaking of the Third World*. Princeton: Princeton University Press.

Espinosa, M. (2009), *Epidemic Invasions: Yellow Fever and the Limits of Cuban Independence, 1878–1930*. Chicago: University of Chicago Press.

Ettling, J. (1982), *The Germ of Laziness: Rockefeller Philanthropy and Public Health in the New South*. Cambridge, MA: Harvard University Press.

Faber, K. (1923), *Nosography in Modern Internal Medicine*. New York: Paul Hoeber.

Federoff, H. J. and L. O. Gostin (2009), 'Evolving from reductionism to holism: is there a future for systems medicine?', *Journal of the American Medical Association*, 302(9): 994–6.

Fee, E. and D. Fox (eds.) (1992), *AIDS: The Making of a Chronic Disease*. Berkeley: University of California Press.

Feudtner, C. (1996), 'A disease in motion: diabetes history and the new paradigm of transmuted disease', *Perspectives in Biology and Medicine*, 39(2): 158–60.

Foucault, M. (1976), 'Historia de la medicalización', *Educación Médical y Salud*, 10(2): 152–69.

Fox, R. C. (1977), 'The medicalization and demedicalization of American society', *Daedalus*, 4: 9–22.

Fox, R. C. (1979), *Essays in Medical Sociology: Journeys into the Field*. New York: John Wiley & Sons.

Garrett, L. (1994), *The Coming Plague: Newly Emerging Diseases in a World Out of Balance*. New York: Farrar, Straus, and Giroux.

Garrod, A. E. (1902), 'The incidence of alkaptonuria: a study in chemical individuality' *The Lancet II*, 160: 1616–20.

Gelles, R. J. (1975), 'The social construction of child abuse', *American Journal of Orthopsychiatry*, 45(3): 363–71.

Gilman, N. (2003), *Mandarins of the Future, Modernization Theory in Cold War America*. Baltimore: Johns Hopkins University Press.

Goffman, E. (1956), *The Presentation of Self in Everyday Life*. Edinburgh: University of Edinburgh Press.

Gould, D. (2009), *Moving Politics: Emotion and ACT UP's Fight Against AIDS*. Chicago: University of Chicago Press.

Gove, W. R. (ed.) (1975), *The Labeling of Deviance: Evaluating a Perspective*. Beverly Hills: Sage Publications.

Gove, W. R. (ed.) (1982), *Deviance and Mental Illness*, Beverly Hills: Sage Publications.

Great Britain Committee on Homosexual Offenses and Prostitution (1963), Report. New York: Stein and Day.

Hacking, I. (1995), 'The looping effects of human kinds', in D. Sperber, D. Premack and A. J. Premack, *Causal Cognition: A Multi-Disciplinary Debate*, Oxford: Oxford University Press, pp. 351–83.

Hall, S. S. (2010), 'Revolution postponed: why the Human Genome Project has been disappointing', *Scientific American*, 1 October.

Hansen, B. (1989), 'American physicians' earliest writings about homosexuals, 1880–1900', *Milbank Quarterly*, 61(S1): 92–108.

Harrington, A. (1996), 'Unmasking suffering's masks: reflections on old and new memories of Nazi medicine', *Daedalus*, Winter, 125(1): 181–206.

Horwitz, A. V. (2002), *Creating Mental Illness*, Chicago: University of Chicago Press.

Illich, I. (1974a), *Medical nemesis: the expropriation of health*. London: Calder & Boyars.

Illich, I. (1974b), 'Medical nemesis', *The Lancet*, 1(7863): 918–21.

Infectious Diseases Society of America (2004), *Bad Bugs: No Drugs: As Antibiotic Discovery Stagnates . . . a Public Health Crisis Brews*. Washington, DC: IDSA.

Jablensky, A. (2009), 'Toward ICD-11 and DSM-V: issues beyond 'harmonisation'' *British Journal of Psychiatry*, 195(5): 379–81.

Jewson, N. (1970), 'The disappearance of the "sick-man" from medical cosmology, 1770–1870', *Sociology*, 10(2): 225–44.

Jones, D. S. (2004), *Rationalizing Epidemics: Meanings and Uses of American Indian Mortality Since 1600*, Cambridge, MA: Harvard University Press.

Jones, D. S. and J. A. Greene (2013), 'The decline and rise of coronary heart disease: understanding public health catastrophism', *American Journal of Public Health*, 103(7): 1207–18.

Jordanova, L. (2004), 'The social construction of medical knowledge', in J. Warner and F. Huisman (eds.), *Locating Medical History: The Stories and Their Meanings*, Baltimore: Johns Hopkins University Press, pp. 338–64.

King, N. B. (2003a), 'Immigration, race, and geographies of difference in the tuberculosis pandemic', in M. Gandy and A. Zumla (eds.), *Return of the White Plague: Global Poverty and the New Tuberculosis*, London: Verso Press.

King, N. B. (2003b), 'The scale politics of emerging diseases', *Osiris*, 19: 62–76.

Klawiter, M. (2008), *The Biopolitics of Breast Cancer*. Minneapolis: University of Minnesota Press.

Kleinman, A. (1980), *Patients and healers in the context of culture: an exploration of the borderland between anthropology, medicine, and sociology*. Berkeley: University of California Press.

Kleinman, A. (1989), 'When you're the one with AIDS, it's a different story', *LA Times*, 26 February.

Klingle, M. (n.d.), *Sweet Blood: Diabetes and the Nature of Modern Health*. Forthcoming.

Knowler, W. C., E. Barrett-Conner, S. E. Fowler et al. (2002), 'Diabetes Prevention Program Research Group. Reduction in the incidence of type 2 diabetes with lifestyle intervention or metformin', *New England Journal of Medicine*, 346: 393–403.

Lamb, S. (2014), *Pathologist of the Mind: Adolf Meyer and the Origins of American Psychiatry*. Baltimore: Johns Hopkins University Press.

Lane, C. (2006), 'How shyness became an illness: a brief history of social phobia', *Common Knowledge*, 12(3): 388–409.

Lane, C. (2007), *Shyness: How Normal Behavior Became a Sickness*. New Haven: Yale University Press.

Latham, M. (2003), 'Modernization', in T. Porter and D. Ross (eds.), *The Modern Social Sciences*. Cambridge: Cambridge University Press, pp. 721–34.

Leavitt, J. (1986), *Brought to Bed: Childbearing in America, 1750 to 1950*. New York: Oxford University Press.

Lerner, B. (2001), *The Breast Cancer Wars: Hope, Fear, and the Pursuit of a Cure in Twentieth-Century America*. Chicago: University of Chicago Press.

Litsios, S. (2015), 'Re-imagining control of malaria in tropical Africa during the early years of the World Health Organization', *Malaria Journal*, 14: 178.

Loscalzo, J., A. L. Barabási and E. K. Silverman (eds.) (2017), *Network Medicine: Complex Systems in Human Disease and Therapeutics*. Cambridge, MA: Harvard University Press.

MacPherson, K. I. (1981), 'Menopause as disease: the social construction of a metaphor', *Advances in Nursing Science*, 6(6): 427–34.

Martin, K. L. (2015), '20 bizarre new ICD-10 codes', *Medical Economics*, 16 June.

McDougall, C. (2012), 'Edward Nahim: Sierra Leone's only psychiatrist', *Newsweek*, 15 October.

McNeil, D. G. (2011), 'Rinderpest, scourge of cattle, is vanquished', *New York Times*, 27 June.

Mizelle, R. (2017), 'Sugar diabetes: medical entitlement and civil rights in America', Colloqium, The Johns Hopkins Department of the History of Medicine, 2 February.

Moynihan, R. and A. Cassells (2006), *Selling Sickness: How the World's Biggest Pharmaceutical Companies are Turning Us All into Patients*. Toronto: Nation Books.

Murray, C. J. L. (2015), 'Global, regional, and national disability-adjusted life years (DALYs) for 306 diseases and injuries and healthy life expectancy (HALE) for 188 countries, 1990–2013: quantifying the epidemiological transition', *The Lancet*, 286(10009): 2145–91.

Newburgh, L. H. and J. W. Conn (1939), 'A new interpretation of hyperglycemia in obsess middle-aged persons', *Journal of the American Medical Association*, 112: 7–11.

Olshansky, S. J. and A. B. Ault (1986), 'The fourth stage of the epidemiologic transition: the age of delayed degenerative diseases', *The Milbank Quarterly*, 64(3): 355–91.

Omran, A. (1971), 'The epidemiologic transition: a theory of the epidemiology of population change', *The Milbank Memorial Fund Quarterly*, 49(4): 510–22.

Packard, R. (2007), *The Making of a Tropical Disease: A Short History of Malaria*. Baltimore: Johns Hopkins University Press.

Packard, R. (2016), *A History of Global Health: Interventions Into the Lives of Other People*. Baltimore: Johns Hopkins University Press.

Palmer, S. (2010), *Launching Global Health: The Caribbean Odyssey of the Rockefeller Foundation*. Ann Arbor: University of Michigan Press.

Patel, V. (2003), *Where There Is No Psychiatrist: A Mental Health Care Manual*. Glasgow: Gaskell.

Paton, A. (1974), 'Medical nemesis—three views: "medicalization" of health', *British Medical Journal*, 4(5944): 573–4.

Patterson, J. T. (1989), *The Dread Disease: Cancer and Modern American Culture*. Cambridge, MA: Harvard University Press.

Pear, R. (2016), 'Medicare program takes aim at diabetes', *The New York Times*, 23 March.

Pellegrino, E. (1979), 'The sociocultural impact of 20th century therapeutics', in C Rosenberg and M. Vogel (eds.), *The Therapeutic Revolution*. Philadelphia: University of Pennsylvania Press.

Podolsky, S. H. (2014), *The Antibiotic Era: Reform, Resistance, and the Pursuit of Rational Therapeutics*. Baltimore: Johns Hopkins University Press.

Pollock, A. (2012), *Medicating Race; Heart Disease and Durable Preoccupations with Difference*. Durham: Duke University Press.

Preston, R. (1994), *The Hot Zone: The Terrifying True Story of the Origins of the Ebola Virus*. New York: Anchor.

Rogaski, R. (2004), *Hygienic Modernity: Meanings of Health and Disease in Treaty-Port China*. Berkeley: University of California Press.

Rosenberg, C. (1998), 'Pathologies of Progress: The Idea of Civilization as Risk' *Bulletin of the History of Medicine*, 72(4): 714–30.

Rothman, B. K. (1977), 'The social construction of birth', *J Nurse Midwifery*, 22(2): 9–13.

Royal College of Physicians (1869), *The Nomenclature of Diseases*. London: Spottiswoode & Co.

Salomon, J. A. and C. J. L. Murray (2002), 'The epidemiological transition revisited: compositional models for causes of death by age and sex', *Population and Development Review*, 28(2): 205–28.

Scheff, T. J. (1966), *Being Mentally Ill: A Sociological Study*. Chicago: Aldine.

Schur, E. M. (1971), *Labeling Deviant Behavior*. New York: Harper & Row.

Scott, J. C. (1998), *Seeing Like a State: How Certain Schemes to Improve the Human Condition Have Failed*. New Haven: Yale University Press.

Scriver, C. R., A. L. Beaudet, W. S. Sly and D. Valle (eds.) (1995), *The Metabolic and Molecular Basis of Inherited Disease*, 7th edition. New York: McGraw-Hill.

Scull, A. (2016), *Madness in Civilization: A Cultural History of Insanity, from the Bible to Freud, from the Madhouse to Modern Medicine*. Princeton: Princeton University Press.

Shorter, E. (1998), *A History of Psychiatry: From the Era of the Asylum to the Age of Prozac*. New York: Wiley.

Sicherman, B. (1977), 'The uses of a diagnosis: doctors, patients, and neurasthenia', *Journal of the History of Medicine and Allied Sciences*, 32: 33–54.

Silverstein, K. (1999), 'An influential health nonprofit finds its "grassroots" watered by pharmaceutical millions', *Mother Jones*, Nov/Dec.

Smith-Rosenberg, C. (1974), *The Male Midwife and the Female Doctor: The Gynecology Controversy in Nineteenth Century America*. New York: Ayer.

Sontag, S. (1989), *AIDS and Its Metaphors*. New York: Farrar, Straus, & Giroux.

Specter, M. (2015), 'One of science's most famous quotes is false', *New Yorker*, 5 January.

Spellberg, B. and B. Taylor-Blake (2013), 'On the exoneration of Dr. William H. Stewart: debunking an urban legend', *Infectious Diseases of Poverty*, 2: 3.

Stage, S. (1979), *Female Complaints: Lydia Pinkham and the Business of Women's Medicine*. New York: W.W. Norton.

Stepan, N. (2011), *Eradication: Ridding the World of Disease Forever?* Ithaca: Cornell University Press.

Szasz, T. (1961), *The Myth of Mental Illness: Foundations of a Theory of Personal Conduct*. New York: Delta Books.

Szasz, T. (1971), *The Manufacture of Madness: A Comparative Study of the Inquisition and the Mental Health Movement*. London: Routledge & Keegan Paul.

Temkin, O. (1977), 'The scientific approach to disease: specific entity and individual illness', in *The Double Face of Janus*. Baltimore: Johns Hopkins University Press.

Tomes, N. (1998), *The Gospel of Germs: Men, Women, and the Microbe in American Life*. Cambridge, MA: Harvard University Press.

Tomes, N. (2016), *Remaking the American Patient: How Madison Avenue and Modern Medicine Turned Patients into Consumers*. Chapel Hill: University of North Carolina Press.

Tuchman, A. (2011), 'Diabetes and race: a historical perspective', *American Journal of Public Health*, 101(1): 24–33.

Wailoo, K. (2001), *Dying in the City of the Blues: Sickle Cell Anemia and the Politics of Race and Health*. Chapel Hill: University of North Carolina Press.

Wailoo, K. (2011), *How Cancer Crossed the Color Line*. New York: Oxford University Press.

Waitzkin, H., Wallen, J., and Sharratt, J. (1979), 'Homes or hospitals? Contradictions of the urban crisis', *International Journal of Health Services*, 9(3): 397–416.

Watters, E. (2010), *Crazy Like Us: The Globalization of the American Psyche*. New York: Simon and Schuster.

Webb, J. (2014), *The Long Struggle Against Malaria in Tropical Africa*. Cambridge: Cambridge University Press.

Weisz, G. and J. Olszynko-Gryn (2010), 'The theory of epidemiological transition: the origins of a citation classic', *Journal of the History of Medicine and Allied Sciences*, 65(3): 287–326.

West, P. (1979), 'An investigation into the social construction and consequences of the label epilepsy', *Sociological Review*, 27(4): 719–41.

Winslow, C.-E. A. (1943), *The Conquest of Infectious Disease*. Princeton: Princeton University Press (and second edition, 1944).

World Health Organization (2011), *Collaborative Framework for Care and Control of Tuberculosis and Diabetes* (WHO/HTM/TB/2011.15). Geneva: WHO.

World Health Report (1999), *The Double Burden: Emerging Epidemics and Persistent Problems*. Geneva: WHO.

4. ANIMALS

ACCAA (1979), *Report on the LD50 Test Presented to the Secretary of State by the Advisory Committee on the Administration of the Cruelty to Animals Act 1876*. London: HMSO.

Altevogt, B. M., D. E. Pankevich, M. K. Shelton-Davenport and J. P. Kahn (2011), *Chimpanzees in Biomedical and Behavioral Research: Assessing the Necessity*. Washington DC: National Academies Press.

Anderson, W. (2004), 'Natural histories of infectious disease: ecological vision in twentieth-century biomedical science', *Osiris, Landscapes of Exposure: Knowledge and Illness in Modern Environments*, 19: 39–61.

Anderson, W. and I. R. Mackay (2014), *Intolerant Bodies: A Short History of Autoimmunity*. Baltimore: Johns Hopkins University Press.

Ankeny, R. A. and S. Leonelli (2011), 'What is so special about model organisms?' *Studies in the History and the Philosophy of Science*, 42: 313–23.

Bending, L. (2000), *The Representation of Bodily Pain in Late Nineteenth-Century English Culture*. Oxford: Oxford University Press.

Bernard, C. (1957 [1865]), *Introduction to the Study of Experimental Medicine*. New York: Dover.

Birke, L., A. Arluke and M. Michael (2007), *The Sacrifice: How Scientific Experiments Transform Animals and People*. West Lafayette: Purdue University Press.

Bliss, M. (2007), *The Discovery of Insulin*. Chicago: University of Chicago Press.

Blum, D. (1996), *Monkey Wars*. Oxford: Oxford University Press.

Boddice, R. (2011), 'Vivisecting major: a Victorian gentleman scientist defends animal experimentation, 1876–1885', *Isis*, 102: 215–37.

Bonner, T. M. (1995), *Becoming a physician, medical education in Great Britain, France, Germany and the United States, 1750–1945*. New York: Oxford University Press.

Braidotti, R. (2012), *Nomadic Theory: The Portable Rosi Braidotti*. New York: Columbia University Press.

Braidotti, R. (2013), *The Posthuman*. Cambridge: Polity Press.

Bresalier, M., A. Cassidy and A. Woods (2015), 'One health in history', in J. Zisstag et al. (eds.), *One Health: The Theory and Practice of Integrated Health Approaches*, Wallingford, Oxon: CAB International, pp. 1–15.

Burkhardt, R. W. (2005), *Patterns of Behaviour*. Chicago: University of Chicago Press.

Bynum, W. F. (1990), '"C'est un malade": animal models and concepts of human Diseases', *Journal of the History of Medicine and Allied Sciences*, 45: 397–413.

Cannon, W. B. (1926), 'The Dog's Gift to the Relief of Human Suffering', *Hygeia*, 4: 3–6.

Cantor, D, C. Bonah and M. Dorries (eds.) (2010), *Meat, Medicine and Human Health in the Twentieth Century*. New York: Routledge.

Clarke, A. E. and J. H. Fujimura (eds.) (1992), *The Right Tools for the Job: At Work in Twentieth-Century Life Sciences*. Princeton: Princeton University Press.

Cooter, R. with Stein, C. (2013), *Writing in the Age of Biomedicine*. New Haven: Yale University Press.

Dukelow, W. R. (1995), *The Alpha Males An Early History of the Regional Primate Research Centers*. Lanham: University Press of America.

Endersby, J. (2009), *A Guinea Pig's History of Biology*. Cambridge, MA: Harvard University Press.

Finn, M. R. (2012), 'Dogs and females: vivisection, feminists and the novelist Rachilde', *French Cultural Studies*, 23: 190–201.

Foucault, M. (1989), *The Order of Things: An Archaeology of the Human Sciences*. New York: Routledge.

Franklin, S. (2007), *Dolly Mixtures The Remaking of Genealogy*. Durham: Duke University Press.

French, R. D (1975), *Antivivisection and Medical Science in Victorian Society*. Princeton: Princeton University Press.

Fridman, E. P. (2002), *Medical Primatology History, biological foundations and applications*. London/ New York: Taylor & Francis.

FRS (1884), 'Brain surgery', *The Times*, 16 December, p. 5; col E.

Gane, N. (2006), 'When we have never been human, what is to be done? Interview with Donna Haraway', *Theory Culture and Society*, 23: 135–58.

Garcıa-Sancho, M. (2015), 'Animal breeding in the age of biotechnology: the investigative pathway behind the cloning of Dolly the sheep', *History and Philosophy of the Life Sciences*, 37: 282–304.

Geison, G. L. (1995), *The Private Science of Louis Pasteur*. Princeton: Princeton University Press.

Goodall, J. (1971), *In the Shadow of Man*. London: William Collins.

Gradmann, C. (2017), 'The measure of disease. The pathological animal experiment in Robert Koch's medical bacteriology', in K. Asdal, T. Druglitrø and S. Hinchliffe (eds.), *Humans, Animals and Biopolitics: The More Than Human Condition*, London: Routledge, pp. 101–18.

Guerrini, A. (2003), *Experimenting with Humans and Animals: From Galen to Animal Rights*. Baltimore: John Hopkins University Press.

Hamilton, D. (1986), *The Monkey Gland Affair*. London: Chatto & Windus.

Hanson, E. (2004), 'How rhesus monkeys became laboratory animals', in J. Maienschein, M. Glitz and G. E. Allen (eds.), *Centennial History of the Carnegie Institution of Washington V*. Cambridge: Cambridge University Press.

Haraway, D. (1997), *Modest_Witness@Second_Millennium.FemaleMan_Meets_OncoMouse: Feminism and Technoscience* London: Routledge.

Haraway, D. (2003), *The Haraway Reader*. New York: Routledge.

Haraway, D. (2008), *When Species Meet*. Minneapolis: University of Minnesota Press.

Haraway, D. (2016), *Staying with the trouble. Making kin in the Chthulucene*. Durham: Duke University Press.

Hardy, A. (2002), 'Pioneers in the Victorian provinces: veterinarians, public health and the urban animal economy', *Urban History*, 29: 372–87.

Hardy, A. (2014), *Salmonella Infections, Networks of Knowledge, and Public Health in Britain*. Oxford: Oxford University Press.

Hinde, R. A. (1959), 'Some recent trends in ethology', in S. Koch (ed.), *Psychology: A Study of a Science*, vol. 2. New York: McGraw-Hill, pp. 561–610.

Jasanoff, S. (2005), *Designs on Nature: Science and Democracy in Europe and the United States*. Princeton: Princeton University Press.

Kay, L. E. (2000), *Who Wrote the Book of Life?: A History of the Genetic Code*. Stanford: Stanford University Press.

Kean, H. (1995), 'The 'smooth cool men of science': the feminist and socialist response to vivisection', *History Workshop Journal*, 40: 16–38.

Kirk, R. G. W. (2008), 'Wanted standard guinea pigs': standardisation and the experimental animal market in Britain ca. 1919–1947', *Studies in History and Philosophy of Biological and Biomedical Sciences*, 39: 280–91.

Kohler, R. E. (1994), *Lords of the Fly: Drosophila Genetics and the Experimental Life*. Chicago: Chicago University Press.

Krause, R. M. (1996), 'Mechnikov and syphilis research during a decade of discovery, 1900–1910', *American Society for Microbiology News*, 62: 307–10.

Lansbury, C. (1985), *The Old Brown Dog Women, Workers, and Vivisection in Edwardian England*. Madison: University of Wisconsin Press.

Lederer, S. E. (1992), 'Political animals: the shaping of biomedical research literature in twentieth-century America', *Isis*, 83: 61–79.

Lederer, S. E. (1997), *Subjected to Science Human Experimentation in America before the Second World War*. Baltimore: Johns Hopkins University Press.

Lederer, S. E. (2002), 'Animal parts/human bodies: organic transplantation in early twentieth-century America', in A. N. H. Creagar and W. Chester Jordan, *The Animal-Human Boundary*, Rochester: University of Rochester Press, pp. 305–29.

Lederman, M. and R. M. Burian (1993), 'The right organism for the job', *Journal of the History of Biology*, 26: 351–67.

Lorenz, K. (1952), *King Solomon's Ring*. London: Methuen.

MacCormac, W. (ed.) (1881), *Transactions of the Seventh Session of the International Medical Congress volume 1*. London: J. W. Kolckmann.

Morris, D. (1962), 'Occupational therapy for Captive Animals', in W. Lane-Petter, *Laboratory Animals Centre Collected Papers vol 11*, London: MRC, pp. 37–42.

Morris, D. (1968), *The Naked Ape*. London: Corgi.

Nathoo, A. (2009), *Hearts Exposed: Transplants and the Media in 1960s Britain*. Basingstoke: Palgrave Macmillan.

Pemberton, S. (2003), 'Canine Technologies, Model Patients the historical production of haemophiliac dogs in American biomedicine', in S. Schrepfer and P. Scranton (eds.), *Industrializing Organisms: Introducing Evolutionary History*, London: Routledge, pp. 191–213.

Pfeffer, N. (2010), 'How abattoir "biotrash" connected the social worlds of the university laboratory and disassembly line', in Cantor et. al., *Medicine and Human Health in the Twentieth Century*, London: Pickering & Chatto, pp. 63–75.

Porter, R. (1993), 'Man, animals and medicine at the time of the founding of the Royal Veterinary College', in A. R. Mitchell (ed.) *The Advancement of the Veterinary Sciences volume 3 History of the Healing Professions Parallels between Veterinary and Medical History*, Wallingford, Oxon: CAB. International, pp. 19–30.

Rader, K. (2004), *Making Mice: Standardising Animals for American Biomedical Research, 1900–1955*. Princeton: Princeton University Press.

Ramsden, E. (2011), 'From rodent utopia to urban hell: population, pathology, and the crowded rats of NIMH', *Isis*, 102: 659–88.

Ridley, R. M. and H. F. Baker (1998), *Fatal Protein: The Story of CJD, BSE, and Other Prion Diseases*. Oxford: Oxford University Press.

Romanes, G. (1888), *Animal Intelligence*. New York: D. Appleton.

Ross, K. D. (2015), 'Recruiting "friends of medical progress": evolving tactics in the Defence of animal experimentation, 1910s and 1920s', *Journal of the History of Medicine and Allied Sciences*, 70: 365–93.

Rossiianov, K. (2002), 'Beyond species: Il'ya Ivanov and his experiments on cross-breeding humans with anthropoid apes', *Science in Context*, 15: 277–316.

Rupke, N. A. (ed.) (1987), *Vivisection in Historical Perspective*. London: Routledge.

Saunders, L. Z. (2000), 'Virchow's contributions to veterinary medicine: celebrated then, forgotten now', *Veterinary Pathology*, 37: 199–207.

Schiller, J. (1967), 'Claude Bernard and Vivisection', *Journal of the History of Medicine and Allied Sciences*, 22: 246–60.

Schwabe, C. W. (1964), *Veterinary Medicine and Human Health*. Baltimore: Williams & Wilkins.

Schwabe, C. W. (1993), 'Interactions between human and veterinary medicine: past, present and future', A. R. Mitchell (ed.) *The Advancement of the Veterinary Sciences volume 3 History of the Healing Professions Parallels between Veterinary and Medical History*, Wallingford, Oxon: CAB International, pp. 119–33.

Schwerin, A. von, H. Stoff and B. Wahrig (eds.) (2016), *Biologics, A History of Agents Made From Living Organisms in the Twentieth Century*. London: Routledge.

Sharp, P. M. and B. H. Hahn (2012), 'Origins of HIV and the AIDS pandemic', *Cold Spring Harbor Perspective on Medicine*, 1: 1–22.

Swabe, J. (1999), *Animals, Disease and Human Society: Human-animal Relations and the Rise of Veterinary Medicine*. London: Routledge.

Thwaites, T. (2016), *GoatMan: How I Took a Holiday from Being Human*. New York: Princeton Architectural Press.

Turner, J. (1980), *Reckoning with the Beast: Animals, Pain and Humanity in the Victorian Mind*. Baltimore: Johns Hopkins Press.

Vicedo, M. (2013), *The Nature and Nurture of Love From imprinting to attachment in Cold War America*. Chicago: University of Chicago Press.

Wells, H. G. (1975[1896]), *The Island of Doctor Moreau*. London: Pan.

Wilkinson, L. (1992), *Animals and Disease*. Cambridge: Cambridge University Press.

Wilmut, I., K. Cambell and C. Tudge (2000), *The Second Creation Dolly and the Age of Biological Control*. Cambridge, MA: Harvard University Press.

Yerkes, R. M. (1925), *Almost Human*. New York and London: The Century Company.

Yerkes, R. M. (1943), *Chimpanzees A Laboratory Colony*. New Haven: Yale University Press.

5. OBJECTS

Ackerknecht, E. H. (1967), *Medicine at the Paris hospital: 1794–1848*. Baltimore: Johns Hopkins Press.

Appadurai, A. (ed.) (1986), *The Social Life of Things: Commodities in Cultural Perspective*. Cambridge: Cambridge University Press.

Bachelard, G. (1934), *Le nouvel Esprit scientifique*. Paris: Alcan.

Baird, D. (2004), *Thing Knowledge: A Philosophy of Scientific Instruments*. Berkeley: University of California Press.

Barfield, W. (2015), *Cyber-Humans: Our Future with Machines*. Cham: Springer.

Borck, C. (2018), *Brainwaves: A Cultural History of Electroencephalography*. New York: Routledge.

Borck, C. (2007), 'Communicating the Modern Body: Fritz Kahn's Popular Images of Human Physiology as an Industrialized World', *Canadian Journal of Communication*, 32(4): 495–520.

Borck, C. (2012), 'The Human Body Re-Built: Body Montages in the Twentieth and Twenty-First Centuries', in C. zu Salm (ed.), *Manifesto Collage. Defining Collage in the Twenty-First Century*, Nürnberg: Verlag für moderne Kunst Nürnberg, pp. 187–97.

Borck, C. (2016), Medizinphilosophie zur Einführung. Hamburg: Junius.

Brown, S. A. (2015), 'Building SuperModels: emerging patient avatars for use in precision and systems medicine', *Frontiers in Physiology*, 6: 318. doi: 10.3389/fphys.2015.00318.

Burri, R. V. and J. Dumit (eds.) (2007), *Biomedicine as Culture: Instrumental Practices, Technoscientific Knowledge*. New York: Routledge.

Cartwright, L. (1995), *Screening the Body: Tracing Medicine's Visual Culture*. Minneapolis: University of Minnesota Press.

Carusi, A., A. A. Hoel, T. Webmoor and S. Woolgar (eds.) (2015), *Visualization in the Age of Computerization*. New York: Routledge.

Clarke, A. E., L. Mamo, J. R. Fosket, J. R. Fishman, J. K. Shim and E. Riska (eds.) (2010), *Biomedicalization: Technoscience, Health, and Illness in the U.S.*, Durham, NC.

Cochrane, A. L. (1972), *Effectiveness and Efficiency: Random Reflections on Health Services*. London: Nuffield Provincial Hospitals Trust.

Cohn, S. (2012), 'Disrupting images. Neuroscientific representations in the lives of psychiatric patients', in S. Choudhury and J. Slaby (eds.), *Critical Neuroscience: A Handbook of the Social and Cultural Contexts of Neuroscience*. Chichester: Wiley-Blackwell, pp. 179–93.

Collins, F. S. and V. A. McKusick (2001), 'Implications of the Human Genome Project for medical science', *Journal of the American Medical Association*, 285(5): 540–4.

Coopmans, C., J. Vertesi, M. Lynch and S. Woolgar (eds.) (2014), *Representation in Scientific Practice Revisited*. Cambridge, MA: MIT Press.

Daston, L. and P. Galison (2007), *Objectivity*. New York: Zone Books.

Dijck, J. van (2005), *The Transparent Body: A Cultural Analysis of Medical Imaging*. Seattle: University of Washington Press.

Duden, B. (1991), *The Woman Beneath the Skin: A Doctor's Patients in Eighteenth-Century Germany*. Cambridge, MA: Harvard University Press.

Duffin, J. (1998), *To See with a Better Eye: a Life of R.T.H. Laennec*. Princeton: Princeton University Press.

Dumit, J. (2004), *Picturing Personhood: Brains Scans and Biomedical America*. Princeton: Princeton University Press.

Eilers, M., Grüber, K., Rehmann-Sutter, C. (eds.) (2014), *The Human Enhancement Debate and Disability: New Bodies for a Better Life*. Houndmills, Basingstoke: Palgrave Macmillan.

Engineer, A. (2000), 'Wellcome and "The Great Past"', *Medical History*, 44: 389–404.

Epstein, S. (1996), *Impure Science: AIDS, Activism, and the Politics of Knowledge*. Berkeley: University of California Press.

Foucault, M. (1973), *The Birth of the Clinic: An Archaeology of Medical Perception*. London: Tavistock.

Gammeltoft, T. (2014), *Haunting Images: A Cultural Account of Selective Reproduction in Vietnam*. Berkeley: University of California Press.

Gifford, F. (ed.) (2011), *Philosophy of Medicine (Handbook of the Philosophy of Science, vol. 16)*. Amsterdam: Elsevier.

Hacking, I. (1983), *Representing and Intervening: Introductory Topics in the Philosophy of Natural Science*. Cambridge: Cambridge University Press.

Harrasser, K. (2016), *Prothesen: Figuren einer lädierten Moderne*. Berlin: Vorwerk 8.

Harris-Moore, D. (2014), *Media and the Rhetoric of Body Perfection: Cosmetic Surgery, Weight Loss and Beauty in Popular Culture*. Farnham: Ashgate.

Hergott, L. J. (2017), 'Aspects of ending a lifelong dream', *Journal of the American Medical Association*, 317(2): 137–8.

Howell, J. D. (1996), *Technology in the Hospital: Transforming Patient Care in the Early Twentieth Century*. Baltimore: Johns Hopkins University Press.

Illich, I. (1975), 'The medicalization of life', *Journal of Medical Ethics*, 1(2): 73–7.

Jay, M. (1988), 'Scopic regimes of modernity', in H. Foster (ed.), *Vision and Visuality*. Seattle: Bay Press, pp. 3–23.

Jones, A. (1998), *Body Art: Performing the Subject*. Minneapolis: University of Minnesota Press.

Jülich, S. (2015), 'The making of a best-selling book on reproduction: Lennart Nilsson's *A Child Is Born*', *Bulletin of the History of Medicine*, 89(3): 491–525.

Kahn, F. (1931), *Das Leben des Menschen: Eine volkstümliche Anatomie, Biologie, Physiologie und Entwicklungsgeschichte des Menschen*, vol. 5. Stuttgart: Kosmos Franckh'sche Verlagshandlung.

Keating, P., and A. Cambrosio, (2003), *Biomedical Platforms: Realigning the Normal and the Pathological in Late-Twentieth-Century Medicine*. Cambridge, MA: MIT Press.

Kevles, B. H. (1997), *Naked to the Bone: Medical Imaging in the Twentieth Century*. New Brunswick: Rutgers University Press.

Kevles, D. (1985), *In the Name of Eugenics: Genetics and the Uses of Human Heredity*. Berkeley: University of California Press.

Kittler, F. A. (1990), *Discourse Networks 1800/1900*. Stanford: Stanford University Press.

Knoeff, R., and R. Zwijnenberg (eds.) (2015), *The Fate of Anatomical Collections*. Farnham: Ashgate.

Kotowicz, Z. (2016), *Gaston Bachelard: A Philosophy of the Surreal*. Edinburgh: Edinburgh University Press.

Lachmund, J. (1997), *Der abgehorchte Körper: Zur historischen Soziologie der medizinischen Untersuchung*. Opladen: Westdeutscher Verlag.

Laënnec, R. T. H. (1819), *Traite de l'auscultation mediate et des maladies des poumons et du coeur*. Paris: Brosson et Chaudé.

Latour, B. (1986), 'Visualization and cognition: thinking with eyes and hands. Knowledge and society', *Studies in the Sociology of Culture Past and Present*, 6: 1–40.

Lawrence, C. and G. Weisz (eds.) (1998), *Greater than the Parts: Holism in Biomedicine, 1920–1950*. Oxford: Oxford University Press.

Lee, K. (2012), *The Philosophical Foundations of Modern Medicine*. London: Palgrave Macmillan.

Lock, M., A. Young and A. Cambrosio (eds.) (2000), *Living and Working with the New Medical Technologies: Intersections of Inquiry*. Cambridge: Cambridge University Press.

Lynch, M. and S. Woolgar (eds.) (1992), *Representation in Scientific Practice*. Cambridge, MA: MIT Press.

Marks, H. M. (1993), 'Medical technologies: social contexts and consequences', in W. Bynum and R. Porter (eds.), *Companion Encyclopedia of the History of Medicine*, vol. 2. London: Routledge, pp. 1592–1618.

Marx, K. (1990), *Capital: A Critique of Political Economy*. Vol. 1, translated by Ben Fowkes. New York: Penguin.

Messac, L. and K. Prabhu (2013), 'Redefining the possible: the global AIDS response', in P. Farmer, J. Y. Kim, A. Kleiman and M. Basilico (eds.), *Reimagining Global Health*, Berkeley: University of California Press, pp. 111–32.

Mol, A. (2008), *The Logic of Care: Health and the Problem of Patient Choice*. London: Routledge.

Mold, A. and D. Reubi (2013), *Assembling Health Rights in Global Context: Genealogies and Anthropologies*. New York: Routledge.

Morgan, L. M. and M. W. Michaels (eds.) (1999), *Fetal Subjects, Feminist Positions*. Philadelphia: University of Pennsylvania Press.

Nelson, J. (2015), *More than Medicine: A History of the Feminist Women's Health Movement*. New York: New York University Press.

Nikolow, S. (ed.) (2015), *Erkenne Dich selbst! Strategien der Sichtbarmachung des Körpers im 20. Jahrhundert*. Köln: Böhlau.

Nilsson, N. L. (1966), *A Child is Born: The Drama of Life Before Birth in Unprecedented Photographs. A Practical Guide for the Expectant Mother*. New York: Delacorte Press.

Paul, D. B. (1995), *Controlling Human Heredity: 1865 to the Present*. Atlantic Highlands: Humanities Press.

Petchesky, R. P. (1987), 'Fetal images: the power of visual culture in the politics of reproduction', *Feminist Studies*, 13(2): 263–92.

Pfeffer, N. (1993), *The Stork and the Syringe: A Political History of Reproductive Medicine*. Cambridge: Polity Press.

Prentice, Rachel (2012), *Bodies in Formation: An Ethnography of Anatomy and Surgery Education*. Durham: Duke University Press.

Rabinbach, A. (1990), *The Human Motor: Energy, Fatigue, and the Origins of Modernity*. New York: Basic Books.

Rapp, R. (2000), *Testing Women, Testing the Fetus: The Social Impact of Amniocentesis in America*. New York: Routledge.

Reiser, S. J. (1981), *Medicine and the Reign of Technology*. Cambridge: Cambridge University Press.

Rheinberger, H.-J. (2005), 'Gaston Bachelard and the notion of "phenomenotechnique"', *Perspectives on Science*, 13(3): 313–28.

Rheinberger, H.-J. and M. Hagner (eds.) (1993), *Die Experimentalisierung des Lebens: Experimentalsysteme in den biologischen Wissenschaften 1850/1950*. Berlin: Akademie-Verlag.

Sappol, M. (2017), *Body Modern: Fritz Kahn, Scientific Illustration, and the Homuncular Subject*. Minneapolis: University of Minnesota Press.

Saunders, B. F. (2008), *CT Suite: The Work of Diagnosis in the Age of Noninvasive Cutting*. Durham: Duke University Press, 2008.

Schott, H. (1993), *Die Chronik der Medizin*. Dortmund: Chronik-Verlag.

Serlin, D. (2010), *Imagining Illness: Public Health and Visual Culture*. Minneapolis: University of Minnesota Press.

Sobchack, V. (2006), 'A Leg to Stand On: Prosthetics, Metaphor, and Materiality', in M. Smith and J. Morra (eds.), *The Prosthetic Impulse: From a Posthuman Present to a Biocultural Future*, Cambridge, MA: MIT Press, pp. 17–41.

Stanton, J. (ed.) (2002), *Innovations in Health and Medicine: Diffusion and Resistance in the Twentieth Century*. London: Routledge.

Sterne, J. (2003), *Audible Past: Cultural Origins of Sound Reproduction*. Durham: Duke University Press.

Street, A. (2014), *Biomedicine in an Unstable Place: Infrastructure and Personhood in a Papua New Guinean Hospital*. Durham: Duke University Press.

Sunder Rajan, K. (2017), *Pharmocracy: Value, Politics, and Knowledge in Global Biomedicine*. Durham: Duke University Press.

Timmermann, C. and J. Anderson (2006), 'Introduction: devices, designs and the history of technology in medicine', in C. Timmermann and J. Anderson (eds.), *Devices and Designs: Medical Technologies in Historical Perspective*, Basingstoke: Palgrave Macmillan, pp. 1–15.

Timmermans, S.; Berg, M. (2003), *The Gold Standard: The Challenge of Evidence-Based Medicine and Standardization in Health Care*. Philadelphia: Temple University Press.

Usborne, C. (1992), *The Politics of the Body in Weimar Germany: Women's Reproductive Rights and Duties*. Basingstoke: Macmillan.

Vall, R. van de and Zwijnenberg, R. (eds.) (2009), *The Body Within: Art, Medicine and Visualization*. Leiden: Brill.

Waldby, C. (2000), *The Visible Human Project: Informatic Bodies and Posthuman Medicine*. London: Routledge.

Weindling, P. (1989), Health, *Race and German Politics Between National Unification and Nazism: 1870 – 1945*. Cambridge: Cambridge University Press.

Young, J. Z. (1968), *Doubt and Certainty in Science: a Biologist's Reflections on the Brain*. New York: Oxford University Press.

Zylinska, J. (2009), *Bioethics in the Age of New Media*. Cambridge, MA: MIT Press.

6. EXPERIENCES

Anderson, S. and F. Staugart (1986), *Traditional Midwives: Traditional Medicine in Botswana*. Gaborone: Ipelegeng Publishers.

Aronowitz, R. (2009), 'The Converged Experience of Risk and Disease', *The Milbank Quarterly*, 87(2): 417–42.

Aronowitz, R. (2015), *Risky Medicine: Our Quest to Cure Fear and Uncertainty*. Chicago: University of Chicago Press.

Bayer, R. and G. Oppenheimer (2002), *AIDS Doctors: Voices from the Epidemic: An Oral History*. New York: Oxford University Press.

Betran, A. P., J. Ye, A-B. Moller, J. Zhang, A. M. Gulmezoglu and M. R. Torloni (2016), 'The increasing trend in caesarean section rates: global, regional, and national estimates', *Plos One*, 5 February.

Bluebond-Langner, M. (1978), *The Private Worlds of Dying Children*. Princeton: Princeton University Press.

Brotherton, S. (2005), 'Macroeconomic change and the biopolitics of health in Cuba's special period', *Journal of Latin American Anthropology*, 10(2): 339–69.

Cleeland, C. et al. (1994), 'Pain and its treatment in outpatients with metastatic cancer', *The New England Journal of Medicine*, 330(9): 592–6.

Cohen, L. (1999), 'Where it hurts: Indian material for an ethics of organ transplantation', *Daedalus*, 128(4): 135–65.

Connolly, M. (2006), 'Population control in India: prelude to the emergency period', *Population and Development Review*, 32(4): 629–67.

Durbach, N. (2005), *Bodily Matters: The Anti-Vaccination Movement in England, 1853–1907*. Durham: Duke University Press.

Ehrenreich, B. (2001), 'Welcome to cancerland: a mammogram leads to a cult of pink kitsch', *Harper's Magazine*, November: 42–53.

Gammeltoft, T. (2014), *Haunting Images: A Cultural Account of Selective Reproduction in Vietnam*. Berkeley: University of California Press.

Greely, L. (1994), *Autobiography of a Face*. Boston: Houghton Mifflin.

Greene, J. (2008), *Prescribing by Numbers: Drugs and the Definition of Disease*. Baltimore: Johns Hopkins University Press.

Gwatkin, D. R. (1979), 'Political will and family planning: the implications of India's emergency experience', *Population and Development Review*, 5(1), March: 29–59.

Hamdy, S. (2008), 'When the state and your kidneys fail: political etiologies in an Egyptian dialysis ward', *American Ethnologist*, 35(4): 553–69.

Human Rights Watch (2009), *Unbearable Pain: India's Obligation to Ensure Palliative Care*. Human Rights Watch.

Human Rights Watch (2010), *Needless Pain: Government Failure to Provide Palliative Care for Children in Kenya*. Human Rights Watch.

Jain, S. L. (2007), 'Living in prognosis: toward an elegiac politics', *Representations*, 98, Spring: 77–92.

Kaufman, S., P. Miller, A. Ottenberg and B. Koenig (2011), 'Ironic technology: old age and the implantable cardioverter defibrillator in US health care', *Social Science and Medicine*, 72(1): 6–14.

Kelly, F. E., K. Fong, N. Hirsch and J. P. Nolan (2014), 'Intensive care medicine is 60 years old: the history and future of the intensive care unit', *Clinical Medicine*, 14(4): 376–9.

King, L. (2016), 'Hiding in the pub to cutting the cord? Men's presence at childbirth in Britain c.1940s–2000s', *Social History of Medicine*, 30(2): 389–407.

Krakauer, E. (2008), 'Just palliative care: responding responsibly to the suffering of the poor', *Journal of Pain and Symptom Management*, 36(2), November: 505–12.

Leach, M. and J. Fairhead (2007), *Vaccine Anxieties: Global Science, Child Health, and Society*. New York: Routledge.

Leavitt, J. W. (1987), 'The growth of medical authority: technology and morals in turn-of-the-century obstetrics', *Medical Anthropology Quarterly*, 1(3): 230–55.

Leavitt, J. W. (2009), *Make Room for Daddy: The Journey from Waiting Room to Birthing Room*. Chapel Hill: University of North Carolina Press.

Lerner, B. (2002), *The Breast Cancer Wars: Hope, Fear, and the Pursuit of a Cure in Twentieth Century America*. New York: Oxford University Press.

Lin, J. T. and P. Mathew (2005), 'Cancer pain management in prisons: a survey of primary care practitioners and inmates', *Journal of Pain Symptom Management*, 29(5): 466–73.

Lindsay, J. (1991), 'The politics of population control in Namibia', in Meredeth Turshen (ed.), *Women and Health in Africa*, Trenton: Africa World Press, pp. 143–68.

Livingston, J. (2012), *Improvising Medicine: An African Oncology Ward in an Emerging Cancer Epidemic*. Durham: Duke University Press.

Lock, M. (2001), *Twice Dead: Organ Transplants and the Reinvention of Death*. Berkeley: University of California Press.

Lopez, I. (1993), 'Agency and constraint: sterilization and reproductive freedom among Puerto Rican women in New York city', *Urban Anthropology and Studies of Cultural Systems and World Economic Development*, 22(3/4) Fall and Winter: 299–323.

Lorde, A. (1980), *The Cancer Journals*. San Francisco: Aunt Lute Books.

Marland, H. (2000), 'Childbirth and Maternity', in R. Cooter and J. Pickstone (eds.), *Medicine in the Twentieth Century*, New York: Routledge, pp. 554–74.

Mitchinson, W. (2002), *Giving Birth in Canada, 1900–1950*. Toronto: University of Toronto Press.

Mold, A. (2012), 'Patients' Rights and the National Health Service in Britain: 1960s–1980s', *American Journal of Public Health*, 102(11): 2030–8.

Nguyen, V.-K. (2010), *The Republic of Therapy: Triage and Sovereignty in West Africa's Time of AIDS*. Durham: Duke University Press.

Novas, C. and N. Rose (2000), 'Genetic risk and the birth of the somatic individual', *Economy and Society*, 29(4): 485–513.

Okeke, I. (2011), *Divining Without Seeds: The Case for Strengthening Laboratory Medicine in Africa*. Ithaca: Cornell University Press.

Parkin, D. M., F. Bray, J. Ferlay and P. Pisani (2005), 'Global cancer statistics, 2002', *CA: A Cancer Journal for Clinicians*, 55(2): 74–108.

Peterson, K. (2014), *Speculative Markets: Drug Circuits and Derivative Life in Nigeria*. Durham: Duke University Press.

Petryna, A. (2003), *Life Exposed: Biological Citizens After Chernobyl*. Princeton: Princeton University Press.

Proctor, R. (1988), *Racial Hygiene: Medicine Under the Nazis*. Cambridge, MA: Harvard University Press.

Rapp, R. (1999), *Testing Women, Testing the Fetus: The Social Impact of Amniocentesis in America*. Berkeley: University of California Press.

Rivkin-Fish, M. (2000), 'Health development meets the end of state socialism: visions of democratization, women's health, and social well-being for contemporary Russia', *Culture, Medicine, and Psychiatry*, 24: 77–100.

Rodriguez-Trias, H. (1978), 'Sterilization Abuse', *Women and Health*, 3(3): 10–15.

Rosenberg, C. (1992), *Explaining Epidemics and Other Studies in the History of Medicine*. New York: Cambridge University Press.

Scheper Hughes, N. (2006), 'Consuming difference: post-human ethics, global (in)justice, and the transplant trade in organs', in K. Wailoo, J. Livingston and P. Guarnaccia (eds.), *A Death Retold: Jessica Santillan, the Bungled Transplant, and Paradoxes of Medical Citizenship*, Chapel Hill: University of North Carolina Press, pp. 205–34.

Schoen, J. (2005), *Choice and Coercion: Birth Control, Sterilization, and abortion in Public Health and Welfare*. Chapel Hill: University of North Carolina Press.

Sharp, L. (2006), *Strange Harvest: Organ Transplants, Denatured Bodies, and the Transformed Self*. Berkeley: University of California Press.

Singh, A., Ogollah, R., Ram, F., and Pallikadavath, S. (2012), 'Sterilization Regret Among Married Women in India: Implications for the Indian National Family Planning Program', *International Perspectives on Sexual and Reproductive Health*, 38(4) (December): 187–95.

Whyte, S. R. (ed.) (2014), *Second Chances: Surviving AIDS in Uganda*. Durham: Duke University Press.

Yahya, M. (2007), 'Polio vaccines – "no thank you!" Barriers to polio eradication in northern Nigeria', *African Affairs*, 106(423): 185–204.

7. MIND AND BRAIN

Adams, V., M. Murphy and A. Clarke (2009), 'Anticipation: technoscience, life, affect, temporality', *Subjectivity*, 28: 246–65.

Bashford, A. (2013), 'Julian Huxley's Transhumanism', In M. Turda (ed.), *Crafting Humans: From Genesis to Eugenics and Beyond*. Goettingen: V&R Unipress.

Berlant, L. (2007), 'Slow death: sovereignty, obesity, lateral agency', *Critical Inquiry*, 33: 754–80.

Borch-Jacobsen, M. (2009), *Making Minds and Madness: From Hysteria to Depression*. Cambridge: Cambridge University Press.

Borck, C. (2016), 'How we may think: imaging and origin technologies across the history of the neurosciences', *Studies in the History and Philosophy of the Biomedical Sciences*, 57: 112–20.

Bowlby, J. (1969), *Attachment*. London: Hogarth Press.

Brooke, John L. and Clark L. Larsen (2016), 'AHR roundtable: the nature of nurture: genetics, epigenetics and environment in human biohistory', *American Historical Review*, 119(5): 1500–13.

Browne, K. (1967), 'Behaviour therapy in relation to contemporary psychotherapy', *Journal of the College of General Practitioners*, 13(1): 321–31.

Casey, B. P. (2017), 'Salvation through reductionism: the National Institute of Mental Health and the return to biological psychiatry', in S. T. Casper and D. Gavrus (eds.), *The History of the Brain and Mind Science: Technique, Technology, Therapy*, Rochester: University of Rochester Press, pp. 229–56. .

Casper, S. T. and D. Gavrus (eds.) (2017), *The History of the Brain and Mind Science: Technique, Technology, Therapy*. Rochester: University of Rochester Press.

Choudhury, S. and J. Slaby (eds.) (2012), *Critical Neuroscience: A Handbook of Social and Cultural Contexts of Neuroscience*. Chichester: Wiley-Blackwell.

Clark A. (2010), *Supersizing the Mind: Embodiment, Action and Cognitive Extension*. Oxford: Oxford University Press.

Cooter, R. (2014), 'Neural veils and the will to historical critique: why historians of science need to take the neuro-turn seriously', *Isis*, 105: 145–54.

Cooter, R. with Stein, C. (2013), *Writing in the Age of Biomedicine* New Haven: Yale University Press

Crile, G. (1915), *The Origin and Nature of the Emotions*. Philadelphia and London: W.B. Saunders.

Cromby, J., Newton, T., and Williams, S. J. (2011), 'Neuroscience and subjectivity', *Subjectivity*, 4: 215–26.

de Chadarevian, S. (1993), 'Graphical method and discipline: self-recording instruments in nineteenth-century physiology', *Studies in the History and Philosophy of Science*, 24: 267–91.

Della Rocca, M. (2016), 'Histories of the brain: Towards a critical integration of the humanities and the neurosciences', in J. Leefmann and E. Hildt (eds.), *The Human Sciences after the Decade of the Brain*. Chichester: Academic Press, pp. 61–80.

Doidge, N. (2007), *The Brain that Changes Itself: Stories of Personal Triumph from the Frontiers of Neuroscience*. London: Penguin Books.

Dror, O. (1999), 'The scientific image of emotion: experience and technologies of inscription', *Configurations*, 7(3): 355–401.

Dror, O. (2001), 'Techniques of the brain and the paradox of emotions', *Science in Context*, 14(4): 643–60.

Dunbar, D., Kushner, H., and Vrecko, S. (2010), 'Drugs, addiction and society', *Biosocieties*, 5: 2–7.

Engstrom, E. (2003), *Clinical Psychiatry in Imperial Germany: A History of Psychiatric Practice*. Ithaca: Cornell University Press.

Faris, R. E. and H. W. Dunham (1939), *Mental Disorders in Urban Areas: An Ecological Study of Schizophrenia and other psychoses*. Chicago: University of Chicago Press.

Fisher, M. (2009), *Capitalist Realism: Is There No Alternative?* Winchester: Zero Books.

Fitzgerald, D., N. Rose and I. Singh (2016), 'Living well in the Neuropolis', *Sociological Review Monographs*, 64(1): 221–37.

Fuller, S. (2013), *Preparing for Life in Humanity 2.0*. Basingstoke: Palgrave.

Fuller, S. (2014), 'Neuroscience, neurohistory and the history of science: a tale of two brain images', *Isis*, 105: 100–9.

Gauchet, M. and G. Swain (1999), *Madness and Democracy: The Modern Psychiatric Universe*, translated by C. Porter. Princeton: Princeton University Press.

Geroulanos, S. and T. Meyers (2016), 'Integrations, vigilance, catastrophe: the neuropsychiatry of aphasia in Henry Head and Kurt Goldstein', in David Bates and Nima Bassiri (eds.), *Plasticity and Pathology: On the Formation of the Neural Subject*, New York: Fordham University Press, pp. 112–58.

Goldstein, M. (1994), 'The decade of the brain: an agenda for the 1990s', *Western Journal of Medicine*, 161: 239–41.

Gopnik, A. (2013), 'Mindless: the new neuro-skeptics', *New Yorker* (9 September), 86–8.

Hacking, I. (2002), *Historical Ontology*. Cambridge, MA: Harvard University Press.

Hakosalo, H. (2006), 'The brain under the knife: serial sectioning in late nineteenth-century neuroanatomy', *Studies in the History and Philosophy of Biology and Biomedical Science*, 37: 172–202.

Hayward, R. (2013), 'Darwin's changing expression and the making of the modern state' in Angelique Richardson (ed.), *Darwin and the Emotions*, Berkeley: University of California Press, pp. 237–61.

Holmes, M. (2017), 'Brainwashing and the cybernetic spectator: *The Ipcress File*, 1960s cinematic spectacle and the sciences of mind', *History of the Human Sciences*, 30(3): 3–24.

Horney, K. (1937), *The Neurotic Personality of Our Time*. London: Kegan Paul.

Jacyna, L. S. (2000), *Lost Words: Narratives of Language and the Brain, 1825–1926*. Princeton: Princeton University Press.

James, O. (2008), *The Selfish Capitalist*. London: Vermillion.

Janet, P. (1926), *Psychological Healing*. London: Macmillan.

Jaynes, J. ([1976]/1990), *The Origins of Consciousness in the Breakdown of the Bicameral Mind*. London: Penguin Books.

Killen, A. and S. Andriopoulos (2011), 'On brainwashing: mind control, media and warfare', *Grey Room*, 45: 7–17.

Kurzweil, R. (2009), 'Going down the rabbit hole', Good (8 April) https://www.good.is/articles/going-down-the-rabbit-hole (accessed 20 July 2017).

Kwinter, S. (2001), *Architectures of Time: Towards a Theory of Event in Modernist Culture*. Cambridge, MA: MIT Press.

Laing, R. D. (1961), *Self and Others*. London: Tavistock Publications.

Levine, R. A. (2001), 'Culture and personality studies, 1918–1960: myth and history', *Journal of Psychology*, 69(6): 803–18.

Leys, R. (1991), 'Types of one: Adolf Meyer's life chart and the representation of individuality' *Representations*, 34: 1–28.

Littlefield, M. and J. Johnson (eds.) (2012), *The Neuroscientific Turn: Transdisciplinarity in the Age of the Brain*. Ann Arbor: University of Michigan Press.

Marx, K. (1857/1993), *Grundrisse: Foundations of the Critique of Political Economy*. London: Penguin.

Maslow, A. (1970), *Religions, Values and Peak Experiences*. Harmondsworth: Penguin.

Meloni, M. (2011), 'The cerebral subject at the junction of naturalism and anti-naturalism', in F. Ortega and F. Vidal (eds.), *Neurocultures: Glimpses into an Expanding Universe*, Frankfurt am Main: Peter Lang, pp. 101–15.

Monbiot, G. (2016), 'Neo-liberalism is creating an epidemic of loneliness', *The Guardian* 12 October.

Moreira, T. and P. Palladino (2005), 'Between truth and hope: on Parkinson's disease, neurotransplantation and the production of the self', *History of the Human Sciences*, 18(3): 55–82.

Noë, A. (2009), *Our of our Heads: Why You are not Your Brain and Other Lessons from the Biology of Consciousness*. New York: Hill & Wang.

Ortega, F. and F. Vidal (eds.) (2011), *Neurocultures: Glimpses into an Expanding Universe*. Frankfurt am Main: Peter Lang.

Pettit, M. and P. Hegarty (2013), 'Psychology and sexuality in historical time', in D. Tolman, L. Diamond, J. A. Baumeister, W. H. George, J. G. Pfaus and M. L. Ward (eds.), *APA Handbook of Sexuality and Psychology Volume 1: Person-Based Approaches*, Washington, DC: American Psychological Association, pp. 63–78.

Pickersgill, Martin. (2013), 'The social life of the brain: neuroscience in society', *Current Sociology*, 6(3): 322–40.

Pieron, H. (1927), *Thought and the Brain*. London: K. Paul, Trench, Trübner & Co. Ltd.

Pitts-Taylor, V. (2010), 'The plastic brain: neoliberalism and the neuronal self', *Health*, 14(6): 635–52.

Price, J. (1967), 'The dominance hierarchy and the evolution of mental illness', *Lancet*, 2: 243–6.

Rees, T. (2010), 'Being neurologically human today: life, science and adult cerebral plasticity (an ethical analysis)', *American Ethnologist*, 37(1): 150–66.

Rose, N. and J. M. Abi-Rached (2013), *Neuro: The New Brain Sciences and the Management of the Mind*. Princeton: Princeton University Press.

Rose, N. and J. M. Abi-Rached (2014), 'Governing through the brain: neuropolitics, neuroscience and subjectivity', *Cambridge Anthropology*, 32(1): 3–23.

Scull, A. (1993), '"Museums of madness" revisited', *Social History of Medicine*, 6: 3–23.

Scull, A. (2015), *Madness in Civilization: A Cultural History of Insanity*. London: Thames and Hudson.

Segerstråle, U. (2000), *Defenders of the Truth: The Battle for Science in the Sociobiology Debate and Beyond*. Oxford: Oxford University Press.

Shamdasani, S. (2010), 'The Optional Unconscious', in A. Nicholls and M. Liebscher (eds.), *Thinking the Unconscious: Nineteenth Century German Thought*, Cambridge: Cambridge University Press, pp. 287–96.

Shamdasani, S. (2020), *Exploring Transcultural Histories of Psychotherapies*. London: Routledge.

Smail, D. L. (2008), *On Deep History and the Brain*. Berkeley: University of California Press.

Smail, D. L. (2012), 'Violence and predation in late medieval Mediterranean Europe', *Comparative Studies in Society and History*, 54(1): 7–34.

Smail, D. L. and A. Shryrock (2013), 'History and the "pre"', *American Historical Review*, 118(3): 709–37.

Smith, R. (1992), *Inhibition: History and Meaning in the Sciences of Mind and Brain*. London: Free Association Books.

Smith, R. (2003), 'Biology and values in interwar Britain: C. S. Sherrington, Julian Huxley and the vision of progress', *Past and Present*, 178: 210–42.

Smith, R. (2005), 'Does reflexivity separate the human sciences from the natural sciences', *History of the Human Sciences*, 18(4): 1–25.

Smith, R. (2007), *Being Human: Historical Knowledge and the Creation of Human Nature*. Manchester: Manchester University Press.

Stadler, M. (2012), 'The neuroromance of cerebral history', in S. Choudhury and J. Slaby (eds.), *Critical Neuroscience: A Handbook of the Social and Cultural Contexts of Neuroscience*, Chichester: Wiley-Blackwell, pp. 135–58.

Szasz, T. (1973), *The Myth of Mental Illness*. London: Paladin.

Tallis, R. (2011), *Aping Mankind: Neuromania, Darwinism and the Misrepresentation of Humanity*. Durham: Acumen.

Tomkins, S. S. (1963), *Affect, Imagery, Consciousness, 2 vols; i., The Negative Effects*. London: Tavistock.

Toms, J. (2013), *Mental Hygiene and Psychiatry in Modern Britain*. Basingstoke: Palgrave.

Tooby, J. and L. Cosmides (1990), 'The past explains the present: emotional adaptations and the structure of ancestral environments', *Ethology and Sociobiology*, 11: 375–424.

Tuke, S. (1813/1996), *Description of the Retreat*. London: Process Press.

Vidal, F. (2009), 'Brainhood: anthropological figure of modernity', *History of the Human Sciences*, 22(1): 5–36.

Wallis, J. (2017), *Investigating the Body in the Victorian Asylum*. Basingstoke: Palgrave Macmillan.

Weber, M. M. and E. Engstrom (1997), 'Kraepelin's diagnostic cards: the confluence of empirical research and preconceived categories', *History of Psychiatry*, 8: 375–85.

Wheelis, A. (1959), *The Quest for Identity*. London: Gollancz.

Wolfe, B. (1953), *Limbo '90*. London: Secker & Warburg.

Young, A. (2003), 'Evolutionary narratives about mental disorders', *Anthropology and Medicine*, 10(2): 239–53.

Young, J. Z. (1950), *Doubt and Certainty: A Biologist's Reflections on the Brain*. Oxford: Oxford University Press.

8. AUTHORITY

American College of Surgeons. (1931), *Committee on the Treatment of Fractures. An Outline of the Treatment of Fractures*. Chicago: American College of Surgeons.

Baker, R. G. (2014), 'Governance, policy and system-level efforts to support safer healthcare', *Healthcare Quarterly*, 17: 21–6.

Baron, R. J. and C. H. Braddock (2016), 'Knowing what we don't know – improving maintenance of certification', *New England Journal of Medicine*, 375(26): 2516–17.

Berg, M. (1995), 'Turning a practice into a science: reconceptualizing postwar medical practice', *Social Studies of Science*, 25: 437–76.

Berg, M. (1997), *Rationalizing Medical Work: Decision-Support Techniques and Medical Practices*. Cambridge, MA: MIT Press.

Berwick, D. M. (1989), 'Continuous improvement as an ideal in health care', *New England Journal of Medicine*, 320(1): 53–6.

Bolon, S. K. and R. L. Phillips Jr. (2010), 'Building the research culture of family medicine with fellowship training', *Family Medicine*, 42(7): 481–7.

Boston Board of Health (1855), 'Sanitary measures of the Board of Health [Boston], in relation to yellow fever'. Boston: Boston Board of Health.

Cantor, D. (2007), 'Introduction: cancer control and prevention in the twentieth century', *Bulletin of the History of Medicine*. 81: 1–38.

Chamberlain, J. M. (2012), *The Sociology of Medical Regulation: An Introduction*. Dordrecht: Springer.

Cochrane, A. L. (1972), *Effectiveness and Efficiency: random reflections on health services*. London: Nuffield Provincial Hospitals Trust.

Da Silva, G. B. (2014), 'Le développement professionnel continu: une autre approche de l'analyse des pratiques de soins', *Santé Publique*, 26(2): 153–4.

Dauphinee, W. D. (2013), 'An International Review of the Recertification and Revalidation of Physicians', in William C. Mcgaghie (ed.), *International Best Practices for Evaluation in the Health Professions*, London, New York: Radcliffe Publishing, pp. 281–310.

Dommann, M. (2006), 'From danger to risk: the perception and regulation of X-rays in Switzerland, 1896–1970', in T. Schlich and U. Tröhler (eds.), *The Risks of Medical Innovation: Risk Perception and Assessment in Historical Context*, London: Routledge, pp. 93–115.

Dunn, M. B. and C. Jones (2010), 'Institutional logics and institutional pluralism: the contestation of care and science logics in medical education, 1967–2005', *Administrative Science Quarterly*, 55(1): 114–49.

Engelmann, L. (2017), 'The past and present of contested medical authority', *Science as Culture*, April: 1–6.

Flynn, J. M. (2017), 'Towards revalidation in Australia: a discussion', *The Medical Journal of Australia*, 206(1): 7.

Harris, J. (2018), 'Altruism: should it be included as an attribute of medical professionalism?', *Health Professions Education*, 4(1): 3–8.

Healy, D. (1997), *The Antidepressant Era*. Cambridge, MA: Harvard University Press.

Institute of Medicine. (2001), *Crossing the Quality Chasm: A New Health System for the Twenty-first Century*. Washington: National Academy Press.

Jones, D. S. (2017), 'Patients, consumers, and the enduring challenge to medical authority', *Reviews in American History*, 45(1): 128–35.

Kohn, K. T., J. M. Corrigan and M. S. Donaldson (1999), *To Err Is Human: Building a Safer Health System*. Washington, DC: National Academy Press.

Langlois, N. (2017), 'Revalidation', *Pathology*, 49: S22.

Marks, H. M. (1997), *The Progress of Experiment: Science and Therapeutic Reform in the United States, 1900–1990*. Cambridge: Cambridge University Press.

Marks, H. M. (2006), '"Until the sun of science . . . the true Apollo of medicine has risen": collective investigation in Britain and America, 1880–1910', *Medical History*, 50: 147–66.

Mcgaghie, W. C. (2013), 'Evaluation in the health professions', in W. C. Mcgaghie (ed.), *International Best Practices for Evaluation in the Health Professions*. London: Radcliffe.

McPherson, K. and J. P. Bunker (2006), 'Costs, risks and benefits of surgery: a milestone in the development of health services research', *The James Lind Library*. Available at http://www.jameslindlibrary.org (accessed 28 January 2007).

Medical Professionalism Project (2002), 'Medical professionalism in the new millennium: a physicians' charter', *The Lancet*, 359(9305): 520–2.

Merkur, S., E. Mossialos, M. Long and M. McKee. (2008), 'Physician revalidation in Europe', *Clinical Medicine*, 8(4): 371–6.

Noordegraaf, M. (2015), 'Hybrid professionalism and beyond: (new) forms of public professionalism in changing organizational and societal contexts', *Journal of Professions and Organization*, 2(2): 187–206.

Parsons, T. (1949), *Essays in sociological theory*. Glencoe: Free Press.

Peck, C., M. McCall, B. McLaren and T. Rotem (2000), 'Continuing medical education and continuing professional development: international comparisons', *British Medical Journal*, 320(7232): 432–5.

Post, R. E., T. J. Weese, A. G. Mainous III and B. D. Weiss (2012), 'Publication productivity by family medicine faculty: 1999 to 2009', *Family Medicine*, 44(5): 312–17.

Reverby, S. (1981), 'Stealing the golden Eggs: Ernest Amory Codman and the science and management of medicine', *Bulletin of the History of Medicine*, 55: 156–71.

Scallan, S., R. Locke, D. Eksteen and S. Caesar (2016), 'The benefits of appraisal: a critical (re)view of the literature', *Education for Primary Care*, 27(2): 94–7.

Teirstein, P. S. and E. J. Topol. (2015), 'The role of maintenance of certification programs in governance and professionalism', *Journal of the American Medical Association*, 313(18): 1809–10.

Van der Meulen, M. W., B. C. M. Boerebach, A. Smirnova, S. Heeneman, M. G. A. oude Egbrink, C. P. M. van der Vleuten, O. A. Arah and K. M. J. M. H. Lombarts (2017), 'Validation of the INCEPT: a multisource feedback tool for capturing different perspectives on physicians' professional performance', *Journal of Continuing Education in the Health Professions*, 37(1) LWW: 9–18.

Wallenburg, I., J.-K. Helderman, A. de Bont, F. Scheele and P. Meurs (2012), 'Negotiating authority: a comparative study of reform in medical training regimes', *Journal of Health Politics, Policy and Law*, 37(3): 439–67.

Weisz, G. (1988), 'The self-made mandarin: the Éloges of the French Academy of Medicine, 1824–47', *History of Science*, 26(1): 13–40.

Weisz, G. (1995), *The Medical Mandarins: The French Academy of Medicine in the Nineteenth and Early Twentieth Centuries*. New York and Oxford: Oxford University Press.

Weisz, G. (2006), *Divide and Conquer: a Comparative History of Medical Specialization*. London and New York: Oxford University Press.

Wennberg, J. E. (1979), 'Factors governing utilization of hospital services', *Hospital Practice*, 14(9): 115–21, 126–7.

Wilson, M. (1993), 'DSM-III and the transformation of American psychiatry: a history', *American Journal of Psychiatry*, 150: 399–410.

Woolf, S. H. (1990), 'Practice guidelines: a new reality in medicine. I. Recent developments', *Arch Intern Med*, Sep; 150(9): 1811–18.

CONTRIBUTORS

Cornelius Borck is Professor of the History, Theory and Ethics of Medicine and Science, and Director of the Institute for History of Medicine and Science Studies at the University of Lübeck. His most recent book is *Brainwaves: A Cultural History of Electroencephalography* (2018).

Nancy N. Chen is Professor of Anthropology at the University of California Santa Cruz. She is the author of *Food, Medicine, and the Quest for Good Health* (2008).

Jeremy A. Greene is William H. Welch Professor of Medicine and the History of Medicine and Director of the Institute of the History of Medicine and the Center for Medical Humanities and Social Medicine at the Johns Hopkins University.

Rhodri Hayward is Reader in the History of Medicine, and Director and founding member of the Centre for the History of the Emotions, Queen Mary University of London.

Richard C. Keller is Professor of Medical History and Bioethics and Associate Dean of the International Division at the University of Wisconsin-Madison. His most recent book is *Fatal Isolation: The Devastating Paris Heat Wave of 2003* (2015).

Robert G. W. Kirk is Reader in Medical History and Humanities at the Centre for the History of Science, Technology, and Medicine (CHSTM), University of Manchester.

Julie Livingston is Julius Silver, Rosalyn S. Silver, and Enid Silver Winslow Professor of History and of Social and Cultural Analysis at New York University.

Todd Meyers is Associate Professor and Marjorie Bronfman Chair in the Social Studies of Medicine in the Department of Social Studies of Medicine at McGill University.

George Weisz is Cotton-Hannah Chair in the History of Medicine in the Department of Social Studies of Medicine at McGill University.

INDEX